Clinics in Human Lactation

Emotional and Physical Trauma and Its Impact on Breastfeeding Mothers

Dianne Cassidy, MA, IBCLC-RLC, ALC

Emotional and Physical Trauma and Its Impact on Breastfeeding Mothers

Praeclarus Press, LLC
2504 Sweetgum Lane
Amarillo, Texas 79124 USA
806-367-9950
www.PraeclarusPress.com

DISCLAIMER
The information contained in this publication is advisory only and is not intended to replace sound clinical judgment or individualized patient care. The author disclaims all warranties, whether expressed or implied, including any warranty as the quality, accuracy, safety, or suitability of this information for any particular purpose.

ISBN: 978-1-939807-64-9

Dedication/Acknowledgements

For Nathan, Jessica and Brandon, who started me on this journey.

For Sheila, who encourages me.

For Tom, who not only supports me, but also believes in me.

And most of all, for all the amazing mothers and babies I have had the pleasure of working with over the years.

Table of Contents

Chapter 1. Introduction

Breastfeeding has been the preferred method of feeding babies since time began. In the 20th century, breastfeeding had become somewhat of a lost art, and increased acceptance of human milk substitutes had quickly stepped in and claimed their place in the world of infant feeding. Medical professionals have recognized and identified breastfeeding as being the optimal choice for mothers and babies; however, increasing breastfeeding initiation and duration rates have been a constant struggle.

When identifying reasons why women abandon breastfeeding, or refuse to initiate breastfeeding altogether, we need to look at the role emotional and physical trauma plays in breastfeeding. Emotional and physical trauma suffered by women at a young age, during pregnancy, during labor and delivery, or in the immediate postpartum period can negatively impact a new mother's ability or desire to breastfeed her baby. Even when she knows that breastfeeding is the best choice, past abuse, physical trauma, or psychological impairment may impede the mother's ability to initiate or continue with breastfeeding.

Trauma can be a difficult subject to address, especially when it involves a delicate topic, such as birth and breastfeeding. In our desire to advocate for best practice among the mother/baby dyad, we must recognize how trauma impacts breastfeeding for the new mother and baby. Healthcare workers, support persons, and family can be helpful to a new mother who is struggling with breastfeeding. By recognizing when trauma may be at the source of the issue, those working closely with the mother/baby dyad can assist in reinforcing the importance of breastfeeding, while being sensitive to a new mother's concerns.

"The scars you can't see are the hardest to heal." – Astrid Alauda.

Definition of Trauma

Pathologically, trauma is defined as a body wound or shock produced by sudden physical injury, as from violence or accident (dictionary.com, 2014). Psychologically, trauma is defined as an emotional wound or shock that creates substantial lasting damage to one's psychological development, often leading to neurosis (dictionary.com, 2014). Research has discussed the implication of intimate partner violence, sexual abuse in childhood and adulthood, and neglect on breastfeeding initiation and success. These forms of trauma can be considered pathological and psychological by definition. Bodily injury trauma can include physical injury to the mother or baby during labor or delivery. Any of these problems alone can make it difficult for a mother to initiate or sustain breastfeeding. Partner emotional trauma with bodily injury trauma can be especially challenging.

Examples of Trauma

Child Sexual Abuse (CSA)

Child sexual abuse can be defined as sexual contact with a child by force, without consent, usually by someone who is in a position of authority or a caregiver. Sexual trauma is relatively common, affecting approximately 20 to 25 percent of women (Kendall-Tackett, 2007). International studies indicate that child sexual abuse can vary from 6% to 62%, depending on the definition of abuse and methods used (Coles, 2009). For example, penetrative abuse may be considered abuse on a different level than genital contact without penetration. Both are considered child sexual abuse.

Research shows that the majority of women that are victims of sexual trauma are women of lower socio-economic status. Higher rape rates are seen in lower income homes and areas, and the lower the income the higher the rate (Perkins, Klaus, Bastian, & Cohen, 1996). Those with a household income under $7,500 are twice as likely as the general population to be victims of a sexual assault (Bureau of Justice Statistics, 2014).

Breastfeeding practices vary considerably by maternal race/ethnicity, education, age, and income. With respect to race and ethnicity, the proportion of infants to have ever been breastfed was higher among Asian, Hispanic, and non-Hispanic White infants (84.2, 82.6, and 78.4 percent, respectively) as compared to non-Hispanic Black infants (58.8 percent). The proportion of infants to breastfeed was highest among those born to mothers with at least a college education (89.0 percent) as compared to mothers of all other educational levels (U.S. Department of Health and Human Services, 2013).

Rates of exclusive breastfeeding are significantly lower than rates of breastfeeding initiation. In 2007, the parents of only 12.4 percent of children aged 6 months to 5 years reported that their child was exclusively breastfed for the first 6 months of life. The rate of exclusive breastfeeding varied by family income, with 10.6 percent of children with family incomes below 100 percent of the Federal Poverty Level (FPL) being exclusively breastfed through 6 months, compared to 14.7 percent of children with family incomes of 400 percent FPL or above. Exclusive breastfeeding rates have not shown the same improvement over time as have breastfeeding initiation rates, and as with breastfeeding initiation, exclusive breastfeeding varies by a number of demographic and socioeconomic factors, such as maternal age and education (U.S. Department of Health and Human Services, 2009).

Childhood sexual abuse has many short- and long-term mental health consequences (English et al., 2005). The specific consequence that an individual experiences depends on the type, severity, age at onset, frequency, and duration of the abuse (English et al., 2005). Dissociation is a common reaction for women suffering from childhood sexual abuse (English et al., 2005). This may enable a victim to mentally escape from the trauma they are experiencing (English et al., 2005). In the context of motherhood, dissociation becomes a maladaptive characteristic that causes mothers to emotionally detach from their children (Silberg et al., 2003). Vulnerability, fear, and loss of control intertwined with the intimacy of childbirth can resurface memories of past abuse. Browne and Finkelhor (1986) hypothesize that the consequences of child sexual abuse begin with disempowerment, with sexual predators disempowering their victims by disregarding their needs and invading their body space. The anxiety caused by this disempowerment may potentially lead to dissociation. When child sexual abuse survivors become mothers, dissociation becomes a maladaptive characteristic that may interfere with the mother-child relationship (Bowman, Ryberg, & Becker, 2008). As Karl explained in a study done in 2004, "Successful breastfeeding requires an intimate interactive connectedness between a mother and her infant for the mother to interpret infant cues and respond appropriately." These characteristics can conflict with mothers that are survivors of childhood sexual abuse.

Intimate Partner Violence

Intimate partner violence (IPV) is a serious, preventable public health problem that affects millions of Americans. The term "intimate partner violence" describes physical, sexual, or psychological harm by a current or former partner or spouse (CDC, 2014).

More than 20% of women experience intimate partner violence during their lifetime (Cerulli, Chin, Talbot, & Chaudron, 2010). Intimate partner violence can be recognized as an act of physical, sexual, or psychological abuse. This includes physical harm from a partner; emotional mistreatment that may be in the form of yelling, disrespect, and threats; sexual abuse, including sabotaging the use of birth control; and economic abuse in the form of controlling money and property.

One would think that pregnancy would shield a woman from her partner's abusive behavior, but in reality, it may have the opposite effect. Intimate partner violence may result in poor physical and mental health, and impair the victim's decision-making abilities. Women experiencing domestic violence not only have a lower duration rate of breastfeeding, but there may be a higher occurrence of postpartum depression. There have been conflicting studies about domestic violence and breastfeeding in regards to initiation and breastfeeding duration. However, amid mothers who choose not to initiate or sustain breastfeeding, victims of domestic violence are statistically overrepresented (Cerulli et al., 2010).

Birth Trauma

When considering the implications of birth trauma on new mothers and their decision to breastfeed, the results can be dramatically different. Birth trauma is often defined as a physical injury sustained by a baby at birth. Birth trauma should also be recognized as a traumatic experience by the mother, which can cause physical and psychological damage carrying into the postpartum period. An example of maternal birth trauma might be a woman feeling that her wants and needs are being ignored, feeling coerced into procedures, such as induction, or experiencing an unplanned Cesarean section delivery. Of course, any of these circumstances can also result in physical trauma as well. Sometimes, during labor or birth, conditions may arise that are out of the mother's control. Feeling the loss of her birth experience has prompted discussion that this can cause a delay in early bonding between mother and baby. The impact of birth trauma on mothers' breastfeeding experiences can lead women down two strikingly different paths (Beck & Watson, 2008). One path can propel women into persevering in breastfeeding, whereas the other path can lead to distressing impediments that can curtail women's breastfeeding attempts (Beck & Watson, 2008). Although each of these described traumas are very different and carry their own significant destiny, they all have similarities that bring them together.

Often, I have witnessed women that have dealt with several traumas under the same umbrella. This may be when a partner is now abusing a survivor of child sexual abuse, and this abuse is making it difficult for her to receive adequate prenatal care. In turn, this woman may experience trauma during delivery, maybe in the form of preterm birth. This new mother now has multiple traumas that she is trying to process, and breastfeeding may not be a priority for her. The case studies throughout this book will showcase many new mothers who have had to address distressing situations such as this. If providers can learn to recognize when a woman is dealing with an abusive situation, whether it be as part of her past or as part of her current situation, adequate support can be offered early enough to make a difference.

Melissa and Matthew

Melissa was pregnant with her first baby. Melissa attended childbirth and breastfeeding classes, and when she went into labor, Melissa was feeling prepared. However, labor was long and difficult, and she received an epidural and approximately five liters of fluid. Matthew was born by vacuum extraction, and Melissa needed significant repair for a third degree laceration.

Breastfeeding was difficult from the start. Matthew was not able to stay with Melissa skin-to-skin after delivery, and he was not able to go to breast until almost two hours after delivery. Matthew was very sleepy in the hospital and hard to motivate for breastfeeding. Melissa received a lot of help and support while in the hospital, but once discharged home, she was lacking confidence and questioning her ability to continue with the feeds. Breastfeeding was painful, and Matthew's weight gain was slow. By the time Melissa contacted someone to come and help her, she was feeling discouraged, tired, and disillusioned. She had no idea it would be this difficult.

While working with Melissa, I could tell that she was feeling withdrawn, and I was genuinely concerned for her wellbeing. Melissa wanted to continue breastfeeding, but was unsure how. She felt as though Matthew was not doing well at the breast, he was feeding constantly, and she was experiencing pain with the feeds. She expressed her concern that she was doing something wrong, and she felt like a failure as a mother. All Melissa wanted was to be able to feed her baby, and have him be happy and content. I gave Melissa different options for how to feed Matthew, including pumping and offering bottles if this was going to help with painful feeds. Together we made a plan that would work for her, without making her feel as if she were failing herself and her baby.

Several weeks later I received a note from Melissa stating how grateful she was for the support she received, and that breastfeeding was going well. Melissa needed some time to recover from a traumatic delivery. Successful breastfeeding was dependent on the support she received. Being able to address Melissa's concerns and creating a plan that worked for her and gave her the time she needed to adjust made all the difference. This plan included offering some bottles, which is not what I would usually recommend in the early days of breastfeeding, but was what Melissa needed to be successful, and breastfeeding thrived once she had this time.

Chapter 2. Childhood Sexual Abuse

"Child abuse casts a shadow the length of a lifetime" –
Herbert Ward

Sexual Abuse

Research has shown us that women of lower socio-economic status are more likely to fall victim to domestic or intimate partner violence and sexual abuse, either as children or as adults (Kendall-Tackett, 2007). In populations where families are living at or below poverty level, sexual abuse and violence are higher in the home environment, and education level is lower. Research also correlates decreased breastfeeding rates, either breastfeeding initiation or duration, with women living at or below poverty level (Kendall-Tackett, 2007).

Sexual abuse is a subject that tends to smolder under the surface. Embarrassment, fear, mistrust, and dissociation can lead to suppression or denial of abuse. In some situations, the abuse is buried so deep that feelings may reemerge when a woman is experiencing the labor and birth of her child. The vulnerability, fear, loss of control, and intimacy of childbirth can rematerialize memories of abuse suffered long ago.

Adolescent Mothers

Adolescent pregnancy and motherhood has a strong link to childhood sexual abuse. Childhood sexual abuse prevalence among adolescent mothers is close to 50% (Bowman, 2007). Childhood sexual abuse has been associated with a variety of high-risk sexual activities, including increased frequency of sexual encounters, number of sexual relationships, and lower usage of risk-reducing contraceptives (DiLillo, 2001). Adolescents who have been sexually abused as children are more likely to become sexually active at a younger age than those who have not been abused. In addition, sexually abused adolescents were almost three times more likely to report pregnancy than non-abused adolescents (Bowman, 2007). Altered child-bearing patterns have been known to be common among survivors of childhood sexual abuse, with sexually abused females giving birth to their first child an average of a year and a half earlier than nonabused peers (Russell, 1986).

Adolescent mothers are less likely to initiate breastfeeding. If adolescent mothers are able to initiate breastfeeding, their babies are more likely to wean at an earlier age than babies of adolescent mothers who have not been abused (Bowman, 2007).

There are several aspects as to why adolescent mothers who are survivors of sexual abuse may decide not to breastfeed. Breastfeeding requires a close, intimate connection between mother and baby, which may be difficult for a survivor of sexual abuse. For these mothers, breastfeeding may feel intrusive and become a source of anxiety, disconnection, and trauma secondary to the abuse (Bowman, 2007).

> Breastfeeding may require too intimate a connection for adolescent survivors of sexual abuse.

If we step back from the emotional connection breastfeeding initiates between mother and baby and focus on lactation as a hormonal experience, hormones that regulate lactation also regulate sexual arousal (Lawrence & Lawrence, 2005). Oxytocin, a hormone released in the body during sexual intercourse is also released during breastfeeding. A new mother who suffered sexual abuse in her childhood may correlate feelings of sexual arousal with breastfeeding and her past trauma. Vulnerability, fear, loss of control, and the intimacy of childbirth may resurface memories of past abuse.

> Due to oxytocin release, breastfeeding may be correlated with feelings of sexual abuse.

Adolescent mothers with a history of sexual abuse may have a difficult time with trust, emotions, and building relationships with others, also known as intimacy disturbance. Intimacy disturbance and dissociation are mental health consequences that are more likely to influence the feeding decisions of adolescent mothers (Bowman, 2007). Being abused as children, adolescent mothers were often abused by someone they were familiar with or someone they knew well, including family members or friends. This may lead to feelings of betrayal and vulnerability. Anger and hostility towards the women in their life, particularly their mother, may dominate the survivor of childhood sexual abuse. The impression that their mother did not protect them from their abuser is overwhelming. Compared to women who have not been abused, survivors prefer to have as little interaction with their mother as possible.

Parenting

Daniel Stern addresses the concept of the Supporting Matrix Theme in the *Motherhood Constellation*. The Supporting Matrix theme is the support system and influence that a new mother may depend on during her childbearing years. A new mother may reflect on the relationship she has experienced with her own mother, which may have a significant impact on the relationship that develops with her own child.

Parenting may prove to be a challenging skill for survivors of childhood sexual abuse for several reasons. Survivors of abuse are more likely to grow up in chaotic family homes, which deny new mothers exposure to healthy parenting models. Survivors struggle with having the confidence needed to effectively parent their own children, which can be a consequence of years of abuse.

> Due to lack of good role models, parenting may be difficult for abuse survivors.

It may be difficult for survivors of childhood sexual abuse to maintain a proper mother/child relationship. Finkelhor and Baron (1986) have noted that failure on the part of survivors to maintain appropriate relationship boundaries with their own children could increase their children's vulnerability to abuse by a male partner, suggesting one potential mechanism for intergenerational transmission of childhood sexual abuse. New mothers who have suffered sexual abuse at the hands of a family member tend to encourage the independence of children at an earlier age. New mothers may resist the dependency of a new baby, which can lead to feelings of resentment for the breastfeeding mother. The attention, attachment, bond, and dependence that a breastfeeding baby may exhibit could possibly be enough to suffocate the childhood sexual abuse survivor, making it difficult to continue an exclusively breastfeeding relationship.

In a study by Douglas (2000), adult mothers with a history of childhood sexual abuse report higher intimate parenting anxiety levels than other mothers. Intimate parenting anxiety might include activities such as breastfeeding and bathing, and acts of affection, such as kissing. Intimate parenting anxiety and fears of abuse may lead some mothers to emotionally distance themselves from their children, leaving children vulnerable to neglect and abuse (Douglas, 2000).

Depression can be a common consequence for an abuse survivor. Women who have experienced multiple types of abuse are more likely to be depressed. For example, women who may have experienced sexual abuse as a child and who are currently in an abusive relationship with a partner may be more likely to exhibit depressive symptoms than women who have only experienced one type of abuse. Dubowitz et al. (2001) found that when mothers have experienced multiple types of abuse, they were more likely to be depressed and used harsher forms of discipline with their children, resulting in significant parenting difficulties.

> Abuse survivors are more likely to suffer from depression.

Donna – with Tyler and Tanya (Twins)

Donna was 24 years old and pregnant with twins. This would make her fourth and fifth babies in five years. Donna expressed an interest in breastfeeding. The father of her twins was younger and not interested in offering support. He was not the father of her other children. In fact, only two of her children had the same father. Donna was devoted to her children and did not have many support people available to her. During pregnancy classes, Donna mentioned watering down formula with her last baby to make it last through the month.

Donna's twins were born several weeks early and were in the NICU for a week or two. In a 1:1 conversation, Donna admitted that she drank castor oil to induce labor because she just could not go another day being pregnant. She delivered by C-section. Donna did some pumping in the hospital, and did put her babies to breast. The father of the twins came to the hospital to see her and the babies, but didn't interact much with Donna.

After the babies were several weeks old, Donna did not interact much with others. She kept mostly to herself, did not express interest in seeing anyone, and did not leave the house unless it was for a medical appointment for one of the kids.

During one appointment, Donna confided that her mother's boyfriend sexually abused her at the age of 12. Donna told the story in great detail, including the name of the officer that took the report. Donna also remembered that her mother was not supportive of her during this time. After commending Donna for reporting the abuse, Donna also remembered that her mother was not supportive of her during this time. After commending Donna for reporting the abuse, Donna responded, "nothing happened. He's free." Donna reflected that before the abuse, she had been an outgoing young girl who enjoyed school. After the abuse, she became introverted and lost her will to do anything with her life. Donna stated that even though she loves her kids, she knows she would not have had five babies with different fathers if the abuse had never happened.

Donna confided her abuse to me after her twins were born. Donna had always been one who did not spend too much extra time at the center. On this day, my meeting with Donna was impromptu; she stopped into my office after her appointment with our mental health therapist. In the center, the participants are usually involved with multiple programs, and are asked to sign a release during their initial intake appointment, which allows the providers to consult with each other if necessary. I approached the therapist later, thinking that she was aware of what was happening. I was concerned for Donna and felt that she was symptomatic of postpartum depression. Donna's therapist looked at me with an expression of sincere surprise. "Donna has never mentioned abuse to me. She must feel bonded and at ease with you. We need to somehow make this work for her, maybe have you join our sessions if she is comfortable with this idea." Unfortunately, Donna stopped coming to the center after this, and we were unable to go any further. Phone calls to her eventually went unreturned. During her pregnancy, Donna and I had developed enough of a connection that she was comfortable discussing her past trauma. Donna did breastfeed for a short amount of time, but never exclusively. One of Donna's twins experienced some health issues and was quite small, which made it even more difficult for Donna to continue breastfeeding. Donna had very little social support and trusted very few people. It was hard for her to get the help she needed.

Concrete Barriers

Survivors of childhood sexual abuse struggle not only with the emotional barriers to breastfeeding, but with concrete physical barriers as well. Breast and body exposure in the postpartum period may be particularly traumatic, especially for a new mother who viewed labor and delivery as distressing or violating. Women may feel strong sensations as her baby feeds, leading to confusion, mixed emotions, and discomfort - both physically and emotionally. Physical pain, such as uterine cramping caused by the release of the hormone oxytocin and nipple pain from baby's latch, may trigger flashbacks of past abuse. Skin-to-skin contact with the baby may be uncomfortable, also triggering flashbacks of abuse.

Unwelcomed physical contact in the postpartum period may lead the new mother to abandon breastfeeding. A well-meaning health professional, such as a nurse or lactation consultant, may touch the survivor's breast in an attempt to latch the baby, increasing anxiety and loss of control. Lactogenesis II, or copious milk production, will bring an increase in breast size, which may prove to be uncomfortable or painful for the survivor of childhood sexual abuse. Nighttime feedings may be perceived as demanding and undesirable, triggering memories of nighttime episodes of abuse. As breastfeeding babies feed on demand, the abuse survivor may become hostile and feel as if she has lost control of her body. Early weaning may make her feel as if she has regained a sense of power.

> Touching a survivor's breasts when helping her breastfeed may increase her anxiety and loss of control.

Jenna

Jenna was 36 years old when she had her first baby. We met when she attended childbirth classes with her husband. Jenna was determined to have a natural birth, but was concerned because her baby girl was in a breech position. After a successful version, which is a procedure that a provider might attempt to turn a breech baby into an optimal position for a vaginal delivery, Jenna delivered her daughter naturally, following a very quick labor.

Jenna struggled to rebound into motherhood, stating that she felt she was having trouble bonding, verbalizing high anxiety over being able to take care of the baby. Jenna felt that when the baby cried, it was somehow her fault. Because of the quick delivery, Jenna experienced tearing, which made it difficult for her to sit. She found breastfeeding painful, crying out each time the baby latched on. Nipple pain, compounded by uterine cramping, was excruciating for Jenna.

When I saw Jenna at the hospital a day after delivery, she looked defeated. Lying on her side in bed, she looked at me and said, "I feel like I was gang raped." Jenna seemed to respond better to people she knew or already had a relationship with, and the hospital lactation consultants asked me to assist with her feeds since we had bonded before she gave birth to her baby.

The maternity center staff that worked with Jenna was concerned about postpartum depression and her ability to care for her newborn. Looking into her history, I found record of ongoing urinary infections, which can be characteristic of sexual abuse. At a doctor appointment years before the pregnancy, Jenna stated that she was not comfortable during a pelvic exam because she felt that she "did not have control." No one recorded a history of abuse in her medical records, and no one noted asking Jenna about abuse.

I went to see Jenna at home after she was discharged from the hospital. She seemed much better, reporting that feeds were still a bit painful, but felt like things were improving. During the feeding, Jenna's brother called from out of state. After speaking to him for a minute, she asked her husband to handle the call. After a long sigh, Jenna explained that her brother has a "troubled life." She shook her head. "My biological father left when I was her age" Jenna continued, looking down at her daughter who was four days old. "The divorce took years and was messy and mean. My brother never got over it. Things happened that he couldn't protect me from and he never forgave himself for that."

Jenna's initial reaction to labor, delivery, and recovery were characteristic of past abuse. Her medical record did not reflect a history of abuse. Jenna's husband was the most supportive husband and father that I have seen. Whenever Jenna was experiencing pain, she called his name and he was right there for her, talking to her in a low voice and stroking her skin.

Health providers, support people, and others who are involved with the care of a new mother may not be aware of her history of abuse. Survivors may bury their past, only to have familiar feelings of anxiety resurface when they become mothers. Studies indicate that 84-98% of people who have been abused never tell a physician about the abuse (Klaus, 2010).

> Most people (84-98%) who have been abused never tell a physician about the abuse.

Health providers should watch for red flags that may indicate a woman is a survivor of abuse. If a woman has an extensive history of medical or psychological complaints, illness, or symptoms that have gone unresolved or problems with pain, this may warrant further exploration (Klaus, 2010).

A number of adult disorders are known to be associated with childhood sexual abuse, such as eating disorders, substance abuse, chronic pelvic pain, sexual dysfunction, severe premenstrual syndrome, gastrointestinal and urological disorders, migraines, phobias, fear of medical or dental procedures, and discomfort with touch (Klaus, 2010). Control issues, excessive dependency on their healthcare provider, and difficulties bonding with their newborn baby can be signals that there may be a history of abuse.

> Watch for signs of abuse – eating disorders, substance abuse, chronic pelvic pain, sexual dysfunction, severe premenstrual syndrome, GI disorders, urological disorders, migraines, phobias, fear of medical or dental procedures, and discomfort with touch.

Suzanne

Suzanne came to the center when she was in her third trimester. This was her first baby. Suzanne did not have any family nearby. She told us she was from another state across the country. When asked how she ended up here, she told us she had run away from home, and stayed here because she ran out of money. During her transition from home, Suzanne had been abused and sexually trafficked. She met the father of her baby after she arrived in town, and hinted at episodes of abuse with him as well. We did not know if he was involved with trafficking Suzanne, and she did not give us very much information about him.

Suzanne became involved with the domestic violence support group at the center. One afternoon she began to complain about contractions. Staff became concerned that she was in early labor and came to get me to assist. Suzanne was clearly in excruciating pain. She was doubled over, and could barely speak. We called an ambulance for her, just in case. As it turned out, Suzanne was not in labor, but was experiencing some Braxton-hicks contractions. This happened once more when Suzanne was at the center, and this time, we assisted by placing Suzanne in a quiet room, bringing her water, and offering support.

The staff at the center was concerned that Suzanne was unable to handle and manage her pain, and we were not sure how she would cope when she went into labor. When Suzanne finally gave birth to a baby boy, she struggled through labor with limited support and a large amount of medications to help control her pain. I went to see Suzanne after she had her baby, and before she was discharged from the hospital. It was more than 24 hours postpartum and Suzanne was still complaining about her pain. The nursing staff kept Suzanne on a continuous morphine intravenous drip to help keep her comfortable.

In time, Suzanne made an amazing recovery. It took a little while for her to adjust to life with her new baby, but motherhood empowered her. Suzanne attended breastfeeding support groups when she was able, and was proud of the breastfeeding relationship she had established with her son. Suzanne was becoming more open about the abusive relationship that she suffered at the hands of her son's father, and was actively looking for help to break away. We celebrated her successes, making sure she knew how far she had come.

Psychologically, survivors of childhood sexual abuse may struggle with issues of control. Because of the loss of control they felt when abused, relinquishing control, especially control over their body, might prove very difficult. This includes medical interventions, feeling unaware of what is going on around them during labor, not knowing what to expect with delivery, and experiencing pain. The need for control may appear as if the survivor is being demanding and inflexible, may show lack of trust for her care provider, and may include a long and unreasonable birth plan (Klaus, 2010).

Contrary to adolescent mothers, other survivors of childhood sexual abuse may actually be more likely to initiate breastfeeding. A study completed by Prentice, Lu, Lange, and Halfon (2002) notes that survivors of childhood sexual abuse readily initiated breastfeeding; however they were less likely to be breastfeeding after four weeks as compared with women who did not report childhood sexual abuse. It is suggested that women who receive prenatal education regarding breastfeeding and have a strong support system in the postpartum period are more successful with breastfeeding.

Communicating with Survivors

It is imperative that healthcare workers who are working with survivors acknowledge the circumstances in which these women live. The ethical responsibility is significant, and the survivors can find themselves in a delicate state during the prenatal and postpartum period. Trust between patient and provider involves accepting others without judging them. In the situation of childhood sexual abuse, a woman may be afraid of being judged by her situation and she may be embarrassed by her history. Lack of trust between provider and survivor may develop a complicated pattern. Without trust and honesty, a new mother may not be truthful about her abusive past and the concerns she may have regarding her past. This will make it difficult for a provider to advise the best practice of care. This can be defined as veracity, or truth, between patient and provider. In order for the healthcare provider to offer accurate information and support, full disclosure is needed. In the case of breastfeeding and sexual abuse, if a patient does not trust her provider enough to be honest about her past, the provider may try to impose the act of breastfeeding upon this mother, with the intent of doing what is best. In actuality, the best thing for this new mother is to find a provider who is skilled in handling survivors of sexual abuse.

Confidentiality is an important aspect to any relationship, especially the relationship between patient and provider. The survivor must feel comfortable disclosing information regarding the abuse or they will not be as willing to be open with the provider. Women who have experienced trauma in their lives may have a difficult time disclosing their history due to trust issues. When considering breastfeeding, if accurate information is not presented, the proper support may be disregarded. Being able to offer support to a new mother regardless of her past history is an important piece to breastfeeding duration. Survivors may be lacking the confidence and self-worth that breastfeeding requires, and they may lack the ongoing familial support that is needed in the postpartum period.

> To gain trust, a provider should listen carefully and validate a mother's feelings, exploring any concerns she has regarding pregnancy, labor, breastfeeding, and the postpartum period.

A provider can gain the trust of their patient if they listen carefully and validate her feelings, exploring what concerns she may have regarding labor, delivery, breastfeeding, and the postpartum period. When working with adolescent mothers, education is an important part of breastfeeding initiation. Educate expectant mothers about their feeding choices in a non-judgmental manner.

> Educate moms about feeding choices in a non-judgmental manner.

Adolescent mothers with childhood sexual abuse history are likely to have come from a family environment that is chaotic, punishing, deprived, and emotionally dysfunctional (Bowman, 2007). It may be difficult to support alternate feeding choices, but it is imperative to recognize when a woman has reached her limit. Considering a new mother's autonomy, she has the right to decide how to feed her baby. The role of the healthcare provider is to offer the best evidence-based information so the patient can make an appropriate decision. Once the survivor has disclosed information, it is the role of the healthcare provider to offer support, no matter what the decision might be and how the healthcare provider might feel about that decision (Brooks, 2013).

> Once a survivor mom has been educated and made an informed feeding decision, support that decision, no matter what the decision is or how you feel about her decision.

Cecelia and Jason

My husband Tom first introduced me to Cecelia. Cecelia's brother was the victim of gang violence and was murdered several months before we were introduced. Tom was investigating the case and interacted regularly with Cecelia. Tom introduced us because Cecelia was several months pregnant.

This was Cecelia's third baby. Her first baby was born when she was 15 years old, her second baby just a couple years later. She had not breastfed her two older children, and decided that she wanted to breastfeed this baby because it was to be her last. We met face to face. I answered some of Cecelia's questions, and she felt confident calling me when the baby arrived. She was expecting a boy. He was to be born about a month before the trial of her brother's suspected murderer was to begin.

The lactation consultant at the hospital called me the day that Cecelia delivered. Cecelia had given birth to Jason, a healthy baby boy, during the night. I arrived mid-morning. Cecelia was in bed. Jason was in the nursery, and she had not seen him since he was born. I spoke with Cecelia briefly, telling her that I would let her rest and come back to see her later in the day and I would bring Tom with me. Cecelia responded by saying, "Don't make me promises that you don't intend to keep." I reassured her that I would be back.

Returning later that afternoon, Cecelia was in better spirits and she had some visitors in the room with her. Jason was also with her. She disclosed that she had not tried feeding him at the breast yet; she just "wasn't sure." I told her that we could try when she was ready. After her visitors left, Cecelia's mother arrived. Cecelia introduced us, and Cecelia's mother collapsed into a chair at the table and began eating take-out food that she had brought with her, without offering anything to her daughter. Cecelia asked her mother to help her with her hospital gown, and her mother responded, "Have your friend help you, I just sat down and I'm tired."

The hospital lactation consultant called me the next day to say that Cecelia was getting ready to discharge and had still not put the baby to breast. The lactation consultant was concerned because Cecelia seemed so distraught over making a feeding decision, and seemed to be in an emotional turmoil over it. I went to the hospital and sat with Cecelia. Jason's father was also there, offering support in any way possible. He wanted what was best for Cecelia and his new baby. Cecelia made it very clear that she wanted to breastfeed, but she just was so unsure. She was not able or willing to articulate exactly why, just that she was unsure. I showed her how to cup feed Jason, and told her that I could come to the house and help once she went home. Cecelia agreed that with the lack of privacy in the hospital, she might feel more comfortable breastfeeding at home.

Once at home, Cecelia put Jason to breast with my help. Jason latched easily, and Cecelia looked relieved, almost as if she had expected something else with the feeding. I offered her praise and encouragement, answered questions, and assured her that I would be available to her for continued support.

I saw Cecelia a few weeks later at the trial of her brother's murderer. I knew that Cecelia would be there, and Tom was also testifying. Cecelia had questions for me about pumping, and rushed off to feed Jason, who was staying with a sitter during the trial.

Cecelia went on to breastfeed for several months, often telling me that she was so grateful that she had made the decision to breastfeed, and was thankful for the continued support. She went on to encourage others to breastfeed as well, and defended her decision to any family members or friends who questioned her.

I did not know for sure if Cecilia had been a victim of sexual abuse. As mentioned in an earlier section, childhood sexual abuse prevalence among adolescent mothers is close to 50% (Bowman, 2007). Cecilia had her first baby at the age of 15. Cecilia's comment about coming back to see her was characteristic of disappointment that had occurred throughout her lifetime. Cecilia's mother did not respond to her needs, signifying a disconnect in the mother-daughter relationship, which can make it more difficult to bond with her own children. Cecilia's turmoil over putting the baby to breast and citing feeling uncomfortable due to hospital interruption were also potential signs of past abuse. Cecilia's life during this time was emotionally chaotic; her brother had recently been murdered and she would be attending the trial in a few weeks following the birth of a new baby. The baby's father was extremely supportive, and Cecilia needed time to adjust to the changes that were happening. Breastfeeding empowered Cecelia, and she was grateful for the continued support.

Summary

In this section, we examined how sexual abuse experienced in childhood may impact a new mother's decision to initiate breastfeeding or her ability to continue breastfeeding. Women who are survivors of childhood sexual abuse may have difficulty bonding with their baby, struggle with the intimacy that breastfeeding brings, and suffer from flashbacks of past abuse. Childhood sexual abuse survivors are more likely to come from a lower socioeconomic status and have a chaotic home life.

Adolescent mothers are 50% more likely to have been abused as children, and we know from research done by Bowman (2007) that adolescent mothers are less likely to initiate breastfeeding and are more likely to wean in the first few weeks post partum. Parenting can be problematic for abuse survivors. Lack of confidence, poor parent/child role models, and relationship problems may make it difficult for new mothers to maintain an effective parenting rapport with their child.

Trust, confidentiality, patience, and understanding are imperative if a survivor and provider are to develop a healthy working relationship. Donna, Jenna, Suzanne, and Cecelia all struggled to overcome a history of abuse. Each of these women wanted to do the best thing for their baby, but needed help and support to realize their goal.

Chapter 3. Intimate Partner Violence

"Domestic abuse, also called intimate partner violence, is the systematic suffocation of another person's spirit." – Joanna Hunter

Domestic violence, also intimate partner violence, or IPV, is considered a major public health issue, with 25% of women having suffered abuse at the hands of their partner. Including medical care, mental health services, and lost productivity, the cost of intimate partner violence was estimated at more than U.S. $8.2 billion dollars in 2008 (Stampfel, Chapman, & Alvarez, 2010). The Population Information Program and the Center for Gender Equity, two respected research institutions based in Washington, D.C., studied numerous local research projects and produced findings in 1999 that echo the consensus of numerous public health and human rights authorities: around the world, at least one woman in every three has been coerced into sex or otherwise beaten in her lifetime (Murray, 2008). Posttraumatic Stress Disorder (PTSD) is the most common mental disorder among abused women, affecting 33% to 83% of women with a history of intimate partner violence (Stampfel et al., 2010). Childhood and lifetime trauma were found to be related to severe PTSD symptoms in women receiving maternity care (Mezey, Bacchus, Bewley, & White, 2005).

Surprisingly, pregnancy does not negate or diminish the act of violence. Between 4% and 8% of women experience intimate partner violence during pregnancy (Kendall-Tackett, 2005). Abuse during pregnancy has the potential to lead to complications during pregnancy and possible negative birth outcomes. Consequences, such as low birth weight, preterm birth, cesarean delivery, low Apgar scores, and neonatal mortality, have been linked to violence during pregnancy (Stampfel et al., 2010). Intimate partner violence around the time of pregnancy or during pregnancy may limit new mothers' abilities to care for their infants based on partners' jealousy and unwillingness to decrease physical and sexual demands on women during the postpartum period (Silverman, Decker, Reed, & Raj, 2006). In addition to women who experience abuse during the prenatal period, one in 17 women report experiencing abuse before pregnancy as well. Violence is associated with unplanned pregnancy. Violent and controlling relationships may not afford a woman the luxury of using birth control. Once pregnant, increased rates of psychological aggression and sexual victimization were noted (Stampfel et al., 2010). Women who reported experiencing intimate partner violence in the year prior to or during their most recent pregnancy were 35-52% less likely to initiate breastfeeding (Silverman et al., 2006). For those women who did initiate breastfeeding, 41-71% were more likely to wean by the time the baby was a month old (2006).

> Low birth weight, preterm birth, cesarean delivery, low Apgar scores, and neonatal mortality have been linked to violence during pregnancy.

Melisa V.

I was working at a community program, which offered support to inner city mothers who were more likely to experience negative birth outcomes. I was the health educator, working along side a case manager, mental health therapist, and social worker.

Within the first few weeks of my employment, Melisa, the case manager, approached me. "You look familiar," she said to me. I knew that Melisa had two kids, a daughter that she had when she was 18 and a son who was just about three.

Trying to find a mutual connection that would have brought us together, Melisa all of a sudden remembered seeing me at WIC. "You worked at WIC, right?" she asked. "Yes," I responded. I was part of the breastfeeding peer counselor program for several years.

Melisa smiled, "I met you when I had my daughter. I was having problems with breastfeeding and you offered to come over to help. My daughter's father was very abusive and I was ashamed to have anyone come over. I didn't want you to somehow find out." Melisa found it difficult to try and maintain the breastfeeding relationship with her daughter, and stopped breastfeeding.

Barriers to Breastfeeding

Women who are experiencing violence at the time of childbirth may struggle with several barriers to breastfeeding. Support for the new mother can be influential to a mother's breastfeeding success. For the woman who is living in violence, she may be lacking in the support needed to continue breastfeeding because women in abusive relationships are often at a loss for supportive partners. Power and control have long been recognized as theories behind the motivation of violence in intimate relationships. Power and control over a new mother's choices, her decisions, and the influence over what she does with her body may lead to disapproval regarding breastfeeding. Gaining and maintaining control by offering bottles to the baby can potentially sabotage a new mother's breastfeeding relationship with her baby.

> Breastfeeding may be sabotaged because of power and control issues.

Kathy

Kathy came to us pregnant and in crisis. She was married to James, who was 20 years older than she was. Kathy and James were at risk of becoming homeless. This was Kathy's first baby, but not her first pregnancy. What little family Kathy did have lived in the Midwest. Kathy's mother died of breast cancer when she was 12, and Kathy never knew her father. After her mother passed away, Kathy bounced around between different family members, finally leaving home at a young age.

During one of our private sessions, Kathy confided that she had been in several abusive relationships over the course of many years. Kathy claimed that she loved James, but admitted that he could be emotionally abusive at times, calling her names and treating her with disrespect. James was an alcoholic and spent what little money they did have on alcohol, going so far as stealing money from her purse.

Kathy had wanted to have a baby for a long time, and became involved with our pregnancy classes and breastfeeding group. She was interactive and excited about the idea of breastfeeding her baby. Kathy often mentioned her mother, and felt confident that James was going to be a supportive and wonderful father.

When Kathy was about six months pregnant, she called us crying and scared. James had been drinking, they had an argument, and he tried to strangle her. We encouraged her to come to see us right away, so we could help her. Kathy expressed her fear and did not want to go back. She asked for our help in finding emergency housing.

Kathy spent two nights in emergency housing before going back to James. He had called her to apologize, and Kathy felt that she should give him another chance. She still continued coming to groups, sometimes talking about James' disrespectful behaviors.

Kathy gave birth to a baby girl via cesarean section. I went to see her in the hospital and James was not there. Kathy said that he was out getting last minute things for the baby, but she was also concerned that he was out drinking. Kathy had initiated breastfeeding, and was very happy that the baby seemed to be feeding well.

Once Kathy was discharged home, I made a home visit. James was with her. I assisted in helping put the baby to breast, but James was voicing his animosity. It was obvious that James was uncomfortable with Kathy breastfeeding their daughter. I made sure to offer support and asked James why he was unhappy with the breastfeeding. All James would say is that he did not think Kathy was making any milk. Kathy continued to put the baby to breast, but James would immediately give the baby a bottle as soon as Kathy was finished. It wasn't long before the baby was refusing the breast and Kathy was exclusively bottle feeding.

The lack of information that a woman may receive during the prenatal period may have a negative impact on her decision to breastfeed. Women who are victims of abuse during pregnancy are less likely to be consistent with prenatal care, which may leave them uneducated about their feeding choices or where they can receive breastfeeding support.

Inconsistency with prenatal care can happen for several reasons. Domestic abuse is more widespread in areas where lower level education and poverty dominate. Access to high-quality prenatal care may be limited. Physical examinations by medical professionals may expose bruising on the woman's body, leading to questions that she may not be ready or willing to answer. It is not uncommon for the abuser to make it difficult for the victim to seek medical attention for her pregnancy because of the risk that abuse may be discovered. The fear and embarrassment that a violent relationship may be detected is enough to deter a woman from receiving adequate medical care. In addition, missed appointments can lead to gaps in prenatal care and vital opportunities for teaching and passing along information to an expecting mother. Most of the women that I have worked with are aware that medical providers, social workers, community programs, and clinics are required to report abuse when children are involved. A woman may be hesitant to disclose her abuse if she is fearful that her children or her unborn child will be involved in an investigation that may ultimately lead to their removal from the home.

> Mothers may not disclose that they are abused because they are afraid their baby might be taken from them.

Victims of intimate partner violence may also experience psychological consequences, which may play a significant role in a mother's decision to breastfeed or to continue breastfeeding. Jealousy from her partner may contribute to psychological control and lack of support for the breastfeeding mother. This may be especially true if the partner feels as if he needs to compete with the baby. Possession over the woman's body or the idea that the breasts are sexual objects may make jealousy worse.

Susan

I was working in a busy hospital as an inpatient lactation consultant. I was asked by the nursing staff to see a mother who had delivered her second baby. Since she delivered overnight, this would be the first visit with lactation.

Entering the room, I introduced myself and asked how I could help. Susan's husband was there with her. Susan asked for a breast pump. "Sure, Susan, I can have a pump set up in your room. Can I ask if there is a problem with the baby latching or are you having pain? "I asked. Susan shook her head, "I would rather just pump my milk and prefer not to latch the baby. These are for my husband." Susan put her hands to her breasts. "This is how I did it with my first baby and I will do it this way for this baby, too."

Susan was definitive that she would not be latching the baby. Abiding by her wishes, I brought Susan a pump and reassured her that I was available to answer any questions she might have. Susan's nurse asked me why I didn't try and convince her to put the baby to the breast. Susan had already made her decision. I felt it was my ethical responsibility to respect that decision, no matter what my personal opinion was. Once Susan's decision was made, it was my responsibility to assist her in reaching her goals, whether I agreed with them or not.

Stress brought on by intimate partner violence may impact a woman's ability to continue breastfeeding. Stress may become a cycle that interferes with milk production, milk ejection reflex, or both, leading to supplementation with formula and early cessation of breastfeeding. Bad habits that may have ceased during pregnancy, such as smoking, drinking, and drug abuse, may begin to creep back into the forefront when stress becomes too difficult to cope with. Lack of self-worth, disempowerment, and depression brought on by physical and psychological abuse may inhibit a mother's ability to continue breastfeeding. This early cessation of breastfeeding could possibly cause additional depressive feelings and guilt over the choice to bottle-feed (Lau & Chan, 2007).

> The stress of being in a violent relationship may interfere with a mother's ability to make milk.

Intimate Partner Violence and Childhood Sexual Abuse

Childhood sexual abuse affects approximately 20-25% of women and intimate partner violence effects approximately 25% of women. Many of the demographics and social concerns of these two forms of abuse seem to be similar. Like childhood sexual abuse, domestic abuse is more widespread in the areas where lower level education and poverty dominate. Victims of intimate personal violence struggle with the emotional aftermath caused by her abuser, complicating her ability to make educated decisions for herself and her baby. Understanding and acknowledging a mother's feelings of shame, humiliation, and inadequacy related to the violence may help caregivers understand the victim's perceptions that she may fail at breastfeeding (Cerulli et al., 2010). Supporting and affirming a mother's decision to breastfeed may counteract humiliation received from her partner.

Communication between mother and baby is fundamental and significant when developing a nurturing breastfeeding relationship. The way a mother responds to her baby's cues in the first days following birth can determine communication between mother and baby throughout that first year. In order for a new mother to be able to respond to her baby's cues, she must be aware of what those cues are and what her baby may be trying to tell her. Several factors can lead to the disruption of this process. Women who are survivors of childhood sexual abuse and victims of intimate partner violence may experience dissociation and have difficulty bonding with their baby. A new mother may also be unwilling or struggle with responding to her baby's cues if this was an unwanted pregnancy or a pregnancy brought on by violence. Reading her new baby's cues may be challenging for a mother who is struggling to form a bond with her infant. Caregivers can offer support by providing the new mother with an opportunity to talk about labor and delivery, giving her the chance to talk about the birth of her baby and how she feels about breastfeeding. By listening and acting in a manner that is nonjudgmental, a new mother may feel more comfortable voicing breastfeeding concerns and identifying possible solutions (Klaus, 2010).

> A survivor mother may have difficulty reading her baby's cues and bonding with her baby. Caregivers can help by giving her the opportunity to talk about the birth of her baby and how she feels about breastfeeding.

As providers working with women, it is important to recognize when it may be necessary to find a provider who may be more skilled in handling trauma survivors. In healthcare, good communication is essential in building a relationship with a patient and providing accurate information regarding individualized care. Communication between a woman and her healthcare provider is imperative in delivering the best care. From the first meeting, a provider and their patient are building a relationship. Practitioners who attempt to form a warm and friendly relationship with their patients were found to be more effective than practitioners who kept their consultations impersonal, formal, or uncertain (Berry, 2006). Women who may have experienced trauma in their lives may have a difficult time communicating with anyone about their history. When breastfeeding is the topic between provider and patient, if an accurate history is not presented, proper support may be disregarded. Trust is an important piece of communication, and building trust between patient and provider is vital for a positive relationship (Berry, 2006). Trust involves accepting others without judging them. Women who are victims of childhood sexual abuse and intimate partner violence may have come from a lower socioeconomic status, have lower education levels, and may engage in habits, such as smoking and drug abuse. Often I have heard women express feelings of frustration when dealing with a provider who is insensitive or who doesn't take the time to listen to their requests. It is important for women in this population to breastfeed their children. The nurturing bond, health benefits, and empowerment that a woman can experience while breastfeeding is particularly powerful for any woman, especially a young mother who is an abuse survivor. However, it is important to remember that every mother is not able to get past her feelings and accept a healthy breastfeeding relationship with her baby. Exploring options with these new mothers, such as pumping and bottle feeding their breastmilk or combination feeding, may help them to adapt easier. These women should not receive a lower level of care and are vulnerable to the care they do receive. Women who live in areas that are poverty stricken may have limited access to providers, and often are restricted by transportation and education. It is important that they feel confident with their provider.

> Caregivers need to acknowledge that not every mother can get past her feelings of abuse and develop a healthy breastfeeding relationship with her baby. Caregivers need to be nonjudgmental in helping the mother explore feeding options appropriate for her situation.

Concerns and questions about breastfeeding are common among women of any culture. Studies have shown that many healthcare providers do not routinely address women's concerns about breastfeeding, regardless of their ultimate feeding choice (Archabald, Lundsberg, Triche, Norwitz, & Illuzzi, 2011). Meaningful discussions with patients about feeding choices are essential, not only to possibly increase breastfeeding rates, but to strengthen the patient-provider relationship and support mothers' feeding goals (Archabald et al., 2011).

Confidentiality is an important aspect to any relationship, especially the relationship between patient and provider. The survivor must feel comfortable disclosing information regarding the abuse or they will not be as willing to be open with the provider. A woman may trust her lactation consultant or her provider enough to disclose her history of abuse or to confess current abuse. A woman may do this for several reasons. She may choose to confide in a provider because she wants to receive help, she wants to talk with someone about her pain, or she wants to explain why she may choose to discontinue breastfeeding.

> A woman may disclose abuse to her provider for several reasons – she wants to get help, talk with someone about her pain, or explain why she is not breastfeeding.

Another barrier that needs to be recognized is the concern that medical professionals are not comfortable or confident discussing abusive relationships with their patients. In a study completed in 2005, only 21% of primary care residents in their final year reported that they were prepared to talk about intimate partner violence with their patients (Black, 2011). One of the reasons cited for this is the fear that the patient will be offended if asked about an abusive relationship. Contrary to this belief, women have stated that they are grateful for information regarding abusive relationships and are not offended by questions their provider may ask. Women also report a higher level of satisfaction when asked about domestic violence if coupled with a compassionate and nonjudgmental attitude (Black, 2011).

> Women are grateful when their provider asks about abusive relationships, especially if the provider is compassionate and nonjudgmental.

Research shows that failure to ask about abuse is perceived as disinterest, leading to a significant decrease in patient satisfaction with their physician (Black, 2011). Considering that intimate partner violence is prevalent and occurs in 20-25% of women, it is not unrealistic that the provider may have a history of abuse as well. It may be difficult and hit too close to home to discuss an abusive partner with a patient. In a situation such as this, the patient should be referred to someone who can step in and offer assistance that is unbiased.

> Failure to ask about abuse is perceived as disinterest. If the provider is not able to discuss suspected abuse with a client, the client should be referred to someone who can offer assistance.

Providers need to take into consideration the concept that a discussion with their patient regarding intimate partner violence is an opportunity to educate their patient, as well as an opportunity to increase trust and communication between patient and provider. This behavior alone may be enough to initiate the break in the cycle of abuse. If healthcare workers ask patients about intimate partner violence when they are presenting with signs and symptoms of abuse, even a brief encounter is likely to encourage disclosure on the part of the patient, especially if the patient does not feel threatened or judged.

Shondra

Shondra came to us six months pregnant. Her eye was blackened. She had a history of alcohol abuse and did not realize she was pregnant until her second trimester. Shondra admitted to abusing alcohol and drugs during pregnancy, stating that since she was unaware of the pregnancy she had continued her addictive behaviors. Shondra admitted that substance abuse helped her cope with the violence. The father of her baby was several years older and Shondra described him as mean, with a drug problem and a history of forcing former girlfriends to work as prostitutes; fathering children with some of them. Shondra denied prostitution. Shondra was recently hospitalized due to an episode of extreme abuse that almost ended in miscarriage.

This was Shondra's first baby. She reported having a good relationship with her doctor, but Shondra was concerned because her doctor told her that he would have child protective services step in after the baby was born if she did not make a move to leave the father of her baby. Shondra told us that she stayed with the father of her baby, but only because she had nowhere else to go. Shondra denied having a sexual relationship with him at that point. Due to the stress she was exposed to daily, and because she had struggled with alcohol abuse, Shondra confided that she was unable to sleep at night unless she was high. Even though Shondra said that she had not been abusing alcohol since she discovered she was pregnant, she did smoke marijuana daily. Shondra told us that her doctor was aware of her addictions and had assured her that he would "go to bat for her" when she had the baby if she was questioned by child protective services.

I contacted Shondra's doctor, and in talking with him, discovered that she was not necessarily being honest in what she was telling him and what she was telling us. Shondra's doctor admitted that he discussed her future living arrangements with Shondra, but never gave her the green light to abuse drugs during her pregnancy. Shondra did not have many family members or friends that she could depend on right now, and talked about her mother who lived out of state. Shondra had mentioned more than once how her mother abandoned her for a life of drugs when she was younger.

Shondra gave birth to a boy. Shondra was breastfeeding, and although she was obviously proud to be able to give her milk to her baby, she often talked about how the father of her baby belittled her and her son for having a breastfeeding relationship. Shondra came to a breastfeeding support group regularly, willing to share her breastfeeding experience with others.

As time went on, Shondra did not come to the program as regularly as she had when she first gave birth to her son. When she did come in, we noticed that she seemed more anxious and unsettled. After her son was about six months old, we would see Shondra on the streets sometimes, and she mentioned "running errands" to make money. She left her son with friends at least once or twice a week for a day or more. By the time Shondra's son was a year old, his father had gone to jail on felony charges.

Shondra's volatile history with not only her own mother, but also the father of her baby, led to questionable actions and decisions made by Shondra concerning both her and her baby. I am convinced that Shondra was able to maintain somewhat of a breastfeeding relationship with her son due to the continued support that was offered to her through the center. Shondra was also encouraged to attend a breastfeeding support group, which kept her involved with other mothers who had similar concerns, and they looked to her for support since her baby was one of the older babies in the group. This was a new experience for Shondra, and she enjoyed telling the other mothers in the group how she overcame her breastfeeding concerns. Shondra also experienced a bond with her son that she had never thought possible because of her abusive past.

Recognizing the signs of past abuse in a pregnant woman or a new mother can be as easy as listening to what she has to say. Being attentive and supportive, asking questions, and listening can be the difference in the way a new mother responds to her baby. When working with women prenatally, I try to pay attention to how they respond to conversations regarding breastfeeding. The response may be verbal or nonverbal. Even a woman's reaction to bonding with her baby will be enough of a concern that may encourage a provider to dig a little deeper to determine if there is a more serious issue that she is struggling with. When I facilitated pregnancy classes and breastfeeding support groups for new mothers as part of a community-based organization that encouraged healthy pregnancy and parenting for young and underprivileged women, I had the opportunity to get to know these women pretty well. When discussing how important skin-to-skin contact is with a newborn, many would cringe at the thought of having their baby so close and intimate, up against their body. Sherri, who was expecting her first baby in a couple of months, looked disgusted when I encouraged that her baby should be placed skin-to-skin with her as soon as he was born. Trying to find out what Sherri was thinking, I said, *"Sherri, is this the first time you heard about skin-to-skin after delivery?"* Her response was, *"There is no way I am touching the baby as soon as he is born. They can clean him up and give him to his father."*

> When a pregnant mother responds negatively to bonding with her baby, it is a red flag to dig a little deeper to determine if she is dealing with a more serious issue.

This response made my mind turn in several directions. Unfortunately, it was a response that I would come to hear often from many other expectant mothers. Was Sherri abused when she was younger? Is Sherri a victim of abuse now, and this is an unwanted pregnancy keeping her from being able to bond with this baby? Of course, it is possible that Sherri has not been subject to any abuse at all; however, her response was so passionate and definitive that I felt the need to look further into her history.

Tamara

Tamara was pregnant with her second baby. She lived with the father of her baby, and the relationship was explosive at times due to Tamara's anger issues. Her first baby, a girl, was only about a year old when Tamara found out about this pregnancy. Tamara and her boyfriend both struggled with substance abuse issues on and off. Tamara's mother was also a bit controlling, and threatened to take the children away from Tamara and raise them herself. There were several complaints to child protective services, including active drug use in front of young children and neglect. Tamara started to attend breastfeeding support group meetings when she was in her second trimester. Tamara was very outspoken and enjoyed the attention she received from comments that she made during class and group settings. During this class, we were talking about concerns new mothers may have about initiating breastfeeding.

"I tried breastfeeding with my daughter," Tamara said. "But I didn't do it for very long. Only a couple of times."

"Tamara can you tell us what happened? Were you feeling pain? Did you have questions?" I asked, trying to understand what Tamara was trying to say.

"It was just weird. I don't know – uncomfortable but not painful. I don't really know why."

Tamara couldn't articulate why breastfeeding was difficult for her, just that it didn't feel right and she didn't know why. For someone like Tamara, breastfeeding could encourage the bond needed for her to be able to be more attentive to her children and, hopefully, see the importance of limiting drug use.

Tamara gave birth to another girl and did initiate breastfeeding after she was born. She continued to come to breastfeeding support, and continued to breastfeed into the first several weeks. I was proud of her for initiating breastfeeding, and I could tell from her comments and from the lack of support from her family that breastfeeding was the complete opposite of what she was "supposed" to do. She slowly started to incorporate more bottles, stating that her mother and the father of her baby were both pressuring her. Breastfeeding dwindled.

Tamara thrived from the attention and support, and I am sure that if we were not able to offer her continued support, she would not have breastfed at all.

It has been my experience that sometimes a new mother isn't aware of why she is uncomfortable with the concept of breastfeeding. Maybe it isn't breastfeeding that is the problem, but the intimacy that breastfeeding provides. A survivor can struggle with the idea that this new baby is completely dependent on her, and breastfeeding encourages a bond like no other. Learning how to share your body with another, even when it is your own child, can be challenging for a survivor to accept.

> Sometimes mothers are not aware of why they are uncomfortable with the concept of breastfeeding. The discomfort may be caused by the intimacy of breastfeeding. Learning to share their body, even with a baby, can be challenging for a survivor.

Summary

Like sexual abuse, intimate partner violence can sway a mother's decision to breastfeed her baby. Childhood sexual abuse and intimate partner violence can be linked in several ways. Childhood sexual abuse affects approximately 20% of the population of women where intimate partner violence may affect 25% of the population of women. Childhood sexual abuse and intimate partner violence have a stronger influence on those who struggle with the same social issues and are from the same lower income demographic. Where lower education and higher poverty are more widespread, childhood sexual abuse and intimate partner violence are known to be more prevalent.

Intimate partner violence has been linked to poor prenatal care, possibly because women in an abusive relationship are fearful of having the abuse discovered through medical examination. Violence during pregnancy is not uncommon and can be blamed for pregnancy complications, including premature labor and delivery.

Stress brought on by intimate partner violence can hinder breastfeeding success because of stress, fear of violence, control issues, and negative behaviors, such as alcohol or drug use. Pregnancy brought on by violence and control from an intimate partner can make it difficult for a new mother to be accepting of her baby and be able to initiate a bond after delivery which would encourage a healthy relationship between the mother/baby dyad.

Providers working with families where intimate partner violence is suspected should be considerate and cautious with how they proceed. Women who are living in violence are in a delicate situation where they are trying to balance what is best for them in a way that will help them stay safe. Women who do not feel judged about their relationship are more likely to be accepting of help and support when it's offered.

> Women living in violent situations are trying to keep themselves safe. When health providers are nonjudgmental, they are more likely to accept help and support.

Chapter 4. Birth Trauma - Baby

"All anxiety goes back originally to the anxiety of birth." –
Sigmund Freud

As mentioned in previous chapters, physical trauma can be defined as physical injury. Therefore, we can define infant birth trauma as being a physical injury sustained by a baby at birth. When considering birth trauma, we must also study the physical and psychological damage that may influence the new mother in the postpartum period and beyond.

Birth trauma can be viewed in many forms. Delivery type and labor stress are just two such examples. In a study by Dewey (2001), it was reported that delayed lactogenesis, or copious milk production, was related to prolonged duration of labor and emergency cesarean delivery (Beck & Watson, 2008). Women who experienced longer labors had elevated stress hormone levels in their blood and lower breastfeeding frequency on the first day postpartum (Beck & Watson, 2008). Prolonged labor may impact not only the mother, but the baby as well. Prolonged labor can be caused by malpresentation of the baby, meaning the baby is not in an optimal position for delivery. Use of anesthesia, such as epidural anesthesia containing fentanyl, may prolong labor. A woman's inability to labor in upright and mobile positions may make it difficult for a baby to move into an optimal birthing station, which is favorable for delivery. This has the potential to prolong labor, leading to operative delivery methods, such as vacuum or forceps delivery.

Implications for Baby

Medicated labor, including induction, augmentation, and pain control, brings concerns for the breastfeeding mother/baby dyad. The induction or augmentation of labor with the use of Pitocin, or artificial/exogenous oxytocin, causes unnaturally strong contractions. The baby is left with less recovery time between contractions and more pressure on the presenting body part of the baby, which is usually the head. This causes more stress for the baby. Powerful and strong contractions may lead the laboring mother to an epidural for relief. As mentioned, this can cause the mother to be less mobile, making it more difficult for the baby to move down, which, in turn, prolongs labor (Smith, 2010). Maternal fever is not an uncommon side effect to epidural anesthesia. Maternal fever is dose related to the duration of the epidural, which is also associated with infant fever, and may lead to mother and baby separation after birth (Smith, 2010).

> Pitocin causes unnaturally strong contractions, resulting in more stress for the baby.

Prolonged labor can have a profound effect on the breastfeeding infant. Torticollis is caused by the shortening or spasm of the sternocleidomastoid muscle (SMC) or is associated with nerve entrapment from cranial asymmetry. Torticollis at birth can be related to intrauterine constriction or position. Babies who are struggling to breastfeed with torticollis may only be able to feed in one position or in restricted positions. Torticollis may adversely affect suck-swallow-breathe and coordinated breastfeeding due to compromised nerves and muscles (Smith, 2010).

> Prolonged labor can cause the baby to have torticollis, which may adversely affect the baby's ability to coordinate the suck-swallow-breathe reflexes needed to successfully breastfeed.

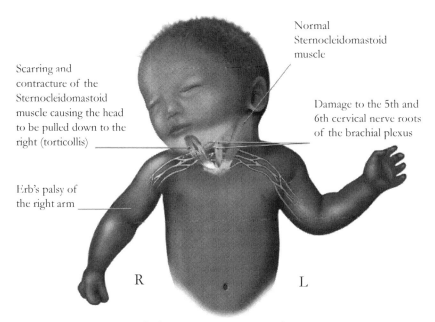

Normal Sternocleidomastoid muscle

Scarring and contracture of the Sternocleidomastoid muscle causing the head to be pulled down to the right (torticollis)

Damage to the 5th and 6th cervical nerve roots of the brachial plexus

Erb's palsy of the right arm

R   L

Baby as seen at 2 months

Figure 4.1. Impact of torticollis on infant.
Source: DoctorStock.com Reprinted with permission.

A study done by Chen, Nommsen-Rivers, Dewey, and Lonnerdal (1998) found that longer labors were correlated to higher levels of stress hormones in maternal blood and cord blood, maternal exhaustion, and lower breastfeeding frequency on day one. Longer second stage labor was associated with longer intervals between delivery and the first breastfeed. Stress on the baby that has endured a long labor can lead to respiratory distress, tachycardia, or bradycardia. This may lead to a separation of mother and baby after delivery. Separation is now known to be physiologically and emotionally stressful for both mother and baby. In addition, mother/baby separation has been linked to increased risk of formula supplementation in the early days postpartum. Formula supplementation of breastfeeding has been consistently associated with shortened breastfeeding duration. Women who use formula supplements in the early postpartum period tend to breastfeed for a shorter time than women who do not supplement (Kurinij & Shiono, 1991). Dewey (2001) studied delayed lactogenesis, or copious milk production, also known as "milk coming in." Researchers noted that physical stressors, such as exhaustion or pain, and emotional stressors, such as anxiety, contribute to delayed lactogenesis by inhibiting oxytocin release (Smith, 2010).

> Stress from a long labor can lead to respiratory distress, tachycardia, or bradycardia in the baby. This may result in mother/baby separation, which is stressful for both mother and baby. Separation has been linked to increased risk of formula supplementation and decreased breastfeeding.

As we delve deeper into the varied examples of birth trauma, many of these situations are the result of interventions during labor, which may lead to operative delivery. Operative delivery is when a baby is born via vacuum or forceps assistance due to delayed second stage labor. Vacuum-assisted birth has been linked to a higher rate of jaundice, which can cause feeding issues for mother and baby. Babies with jaundice can exhibit difficult feeding behaviors due to sleepiness, and babies who require phototherapy experience separation from their mother for extended periods of time, increasing stress and the likelihood of formula supplementation. This will limit the ability for mother and baby to feed on demand and establish a positive breastfeeding relationship in the first few days postpartum.

Lauren and Caiden

Lauren called me for breastfeeding help when Caiden was a week old. Lauren was supplementing feedings with formula and using a nipple shield to assist with the latch. Lauren stated that the nursing staff gave her a nipple shield right after she delivered due to flattened nipples.

When I asked about Caiden's delivery, Lauren reported, "I asked for an epidural, but they were really busy, so it took a little while for them to get to me. As they were putting in my epidural, I told them that I felt a lot of pressure and wanted to push. It turned out that I was already about 10 cm, but they didn't check before starting the epidural, so they didn't know that. But I really felt like I needed the epidural. Then I pushed for over two hours and Caiden was born using the vacuum. I had to have an episiotomy. Caiden developed jaundice and went under the lights when he was three days old. He had lost about 13% of his birth weight, and we were supplementing to get some of his weight back. Now the pediatrician suggested that I pump after every feeding and offer a supplement. It's all very overwhelming."

If Lauren had been offered more support throughout labor and had been checked prior to starting the epidural, she may have been able to avoid a medicated delivery that let to an operative delivery with vacuum assistance and episiotomy. When I asked Lauren why she was given a nipple shield, she said that it was to help Caiden latch due to flattened nipples. When I assisted with Caiden's feeding, I observed that Lauren's nipples were not necessarily flat. Lauren did receive fluids to compliment the epidural anesthesia, which, in turn, caused some swelling in the breast tissue and around the nipple. Lauren was overcome with the amount of work she was doing to breastfeed and questioned her ability to continue. Follow-up calls to Lauren went unanswered.

Caput, cephalohematoma, and bruising are related to vacuum-assisted births. Caput is a large swelling on the infant's head caused by the pressure of the wall of the vagina during delivery. The swelling is usually on the part of the baby's head that comes first. Often, we see caput after a prolonged delivery or due to vacuum extraction (www.baby-safety-concerns.com/traumatic-birth-injuries.html).

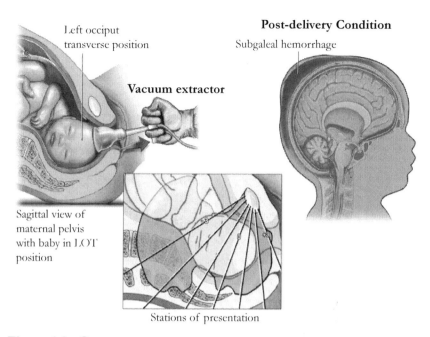

Left occiput transverse position

Post-delivery Condition

Subgaleal hemorrhage

Vacuum extractor

Sagittal view of maternal pelvis with baby in LOT position

Stations of presentation

Figure 4.2. Caput.
Source: DoctorStock.com. Reprinted with permission.

> Prolonged labor can lead to caput, cephalohematoma, and bruising from vacuum-assisted births, making it difficult to find a comfortable position for baby to breastfeed and coordinate suck-swallow-breathe needed for successful breastfeeding.

Lactation and care providers often report that babies with caput feed poorly in horizontal positions and behave as if they have a severe headache (Smith, 2010). Coordination may be adversely effected by instrument-assisted birth because of possible nerve damage. Misalignment, swelling, or disruption of cranial nerves and veins caused by mechanical force may make it difficult for the newborn baby to coordinate suck-swallow-breathe to accommodate successful breastfeeding. Facial asymmetry and facial palsy are also related to operative delivery and birth trauma. Forceps may compromise facial nerves, including sensory fibers to the palate and tongue, causing difficulty for the infant to begin feeding and control facial muscles, lips, and jaw (Smith, 2010). A newborn's inability to grasp the suck-swallow-breathe patterns within the first few days postpartum makes it increasingly difficult for exclusive breastfeeding to become established. When investigating early cessation of breastfeeding, Hall et al. (2002) report that vaginal delivery by vacuum extraction is a significant predictor of breastfeeding problems, which leads to early weaning. Beck and Watson (2008) note that an important component when describing birth trauma include lack of caring and communication by labor and delivery staff, provision of unsafe care, and the glossing over of their traumatic experiences as the delivery outcome took center stage. Additional risk factors for perceiving labor and delivery as traumatic include a high level of obstetric intervention, dissatisfaction with care, loss of control, and history of psychiatric counseling (Beck & Watson, 2008).

Amanda and Baby Nalah

When I met Amanda she was pregnant with her third baby. Amanda had two boys, age five and six, and was expecting a girl. The father of her unborn baby was the father of her five-year-old, but she did not talk about the father of her six-year-old.

Amanda was unsure about breastfeeding her daughter and implied that she did not have a positive experience with her boys. When I asked Amanda about breastfeeding her boys, she admitted that she tried to breastfeed, but was unsuccessful. Amanda reported that her boys "didn't latch" and the nurses kept touching her breast. Amanda found this offensive. Because of this intrusion, Amanda began bottle feeding before hospital discharge. Amanda's first son was born by vacuum extraction and suffered from facial palsy. Amanda was aware that the palsy was caused by operative delivery, stating that the doctor who delivered him told her what happened. Amanda reported that she could still see the palsy in his face six years later, but usually only when he cried. Amanda continued to see the same doctor for her pregnancies and planned to have him deliver this baby. Amanda did not have many choices for medical care due to where she lived and was unsure about changing providers.

When Amanda's daughter, Nalah, was born, she was able to successfully breastfeed with continued breastfeeding support throughout the following months. Even though Nalah portrayed normal newborn behaviors, Amanda was insecure about her ability to trust her instincts because breastfeeding was so different from bottle feeding her sons. Renewed sense of self emerged as Amanda became more comfortable asking for guidance with breastfeeding, and she was able to enjoy a successful breastfeeding relationship for several months.

Often, women who were traumatized, either emotionally or physically, during childbirth feel violated and stripped of their dignity. As a result, some mothers become vigilant about protecting their body from being violated again, specifically the breast. Beck and Watson (2008) found that feeling violated during childbirth impedes breastfeeding. Women want to regain control of their bodies.

Suctioning the newborn baby can cause physical damage to the oropharynx, which, in turn, can cause pain during feeding attempts for the infant, and nipple pain for the mother if the baby is resistant to a deep latch. Babies who experience suctioning may become protective of their airway, pulling back when deep latch is attempted or sliding to the tip of the nipple during the feed after latch on. Nipple damage and nipple pain is one of the most frequent reasons for supplementation in the early days of breastfeeding, and one of the most common reasons for breastfeeding cessation.

> Babies who are suctioned may try to protect their airways and be resistant to a deep latch, leading to nipple damage and pain.

Cheryl

Cheryl was a nursing student doing her maternity rotation. She had the opportunity to observe a primary cesarean delivery. Hearing about the delivery from her point of view was enlightening, because it was the first time Cheryl had experienced anything like this.

"It was a C-section because the baby was in a breech position. It was amazing to see how aggressive they were with the mother. After the abdominal cut was made, the doctor was on one side of the incision, a fellow on the other side, and they just pulled as hard as they could to open the incision. When they got to the baby, the doctor called out that there was meconium. The nurse immediately called for the pediatric team. The body of the baby was out, but the doctor couldn't seem to get the head out. He stuck two fingers into the baby's mouth and pulled, what seemed to be very hard to me, to get the head out. As soon as the baby came out, they gave him to the pediatric team. The pediatric team pulled the baby's head back and stuck something down his throat. I can't remember exactly what it was called, but the purpose was to clear the airway and suction any meconium out.

> After they suctioned, they did all the normal things - temp, weight, measurements, vaccines, vitamin K., etc. and they just kept a close eye on the baby for the next day to see if there were symptoms of meconium aspiration syndrome."

After Cheryl told me about this delivery, my first thought immediately went to breastfeeding. I do not know the results of how the baby fed or what happened after delivery, but this mother and baby should be offered increased amounts of support while breastfeeding becomes established.

Medications introduced during labor to induce, augment, or assist with pain management can negatively impact a baby's ability to breastfeed. Epidural use during labor and delivery has become increasingly popular among women over the last few decades. Although its use has become more mainstream during labor and delivery, the consequences of birth with anesthesia has not been seen as a concern. Epidural anesthesia is a regional anesthetic which blocks nerve impulses from lower spinal segments. Epidural anesthesia can be produced using a class of drugs called local anesthetics, such as bupivacaine, chloroprocaine or lidocaine (American Pregnancy Association, 2007). They are usually combined with opioids or narcotics, such as fentanyl and sufentanil (American Pregnancy Association, 2007). Regional anesthesia is injected between the vertebrae in the spine using a catheter. The catheter is then secured to the back until after delivery.

Various research studies examined by Howie and McMullen (2006) support the theory that higher doses of epidural fentanyl are associated with breastfeeding complications. The study reports that 21% of women having breastfeeding difficulties were from a high-dose fentanyl group, but only 10% of breastfeeding difficulties were reported with the immediate and no fentanyl groups (Howie & McMullen, 2006). Women who were identified as being part of the high fentanyl group were also less likely to be breastfeeding at six weeks postpartum (Howie & McMullen, 2006). Jordan, Emery, Bradshaw, Watkins, & Friswell (2005) observed the feeding methods at discharge among women who delivered full term babies in a hospital setting. When asked about feeding choice, women who stated that they planned to breastfeed prior to delivery were 63% more likely to bottle feed if they received fentanyl epidural analgesia during labor (2005). With exclusive breastfeeding rates in the United States at 16% at six months (CDC, 2012), breastfeeding duration is a growing concern.

> Mothers receiving high-dose fentanyl in epidurals had more breastfeeding problems than mothers receiving low-dose or no fentanyl in epidurals.

Henderson, Dickenson, Evans, McDonald and Paech (2003) conducted a study that looked at how epidural use may interfere with breastfeeding duration. Using a randomized controlled trial method, breastfeeding was initiated by 95% of the participants in the study. Women choosing epidural anesthesia received a combination spinal epidural containing fentanyl and bupivacaine. Epidural use in this study was associated with interventions, such as longer labor and induction. By six months, only 40% of the participants were still breastfeeding. Breastfeeding duration was significantly lower in women who received epidural anesthesia than in women who received narcotic analgesia or no medication at all (Henderson et al., 2003). Placental transfer has been noted with the use of both fentanyl and sufentanyl given by way of epidural. Bupivacaine enters the maternal bloodstream rapidly, crossing the placenta (Henderson et al., 2006). Measurable concentrations are present in fetal circulation within 10 minutes of injection (Henderson et al., 2006). These medications target the mothers' sensory nerve tissue, and likely affect the baby's sensory nerve tissue as well, interfering with the newborn's ability to latch and suck. As mentioned previously, epidural anesthesia has been associated with prolonged second stage labor, which can lead to interventions, such as operative delivery and possible cesarean delivery. Oxytocin and prolactin are negatively affected by epidurals, which can interfere with maternal bonding and uterine contractions. If educated about the potential risks a medicated delivery may have on the breastfeeding relationship for the mother/baby dyad, a new mother may be better prepared to watch for breastfeeding problems. Medical staff that is working with new families in the immediate postpartum period should be aware of how to best assist mothers who have experienced a medicated delivery, and how to best protect the breastfeeding relationship between mother and baby.

> Mothers receiving epidurals should be educated about the impact of a medicated delivery on breastfeeding and what to watch for to indicate breastfeeding problems. She should be advised on ways to feed to overcome the problems.

Summary

It has been my experience that birth trauma suffered by the baby can be easily overlooked and misunderstood. Babies affected by birth trauma, whether it is an obvious hematoma as a result of an operative delivery or trauma that is more subtle, such as mother/baby separation, may have problems breastfeeding. To identify birth trauma as a contributing factor to breastfeeding problems, providers and healthcare workers who are assisting the mother/baby dyad must look at the birth history to see what has transpired. Babies that are born after a long labor, operative delivery, such as vacuum extraction, or medicated delivery are just a few indications of when birth trauma may be present. Providers can assist with breastfeeding by offering support to new mothers and offering suggestions to assist with feedings. Ongoing support after hospital discharge can be a strong indicator of breastfeeding success. Recognizing that birth trauma can cause breastfeeding problems is imperative, and women should be educated about how medications and delivery can affect their baby's ability to feed effectively.

> Traumatic birth can affect a baby's ability to breastfeed. After reviewing the birth history, providers should educate mothers on how medications and delivery can affect their baby's ability to feed effectively and offer suggestions on ways to breastfeed to alleviate or lessen the problems caused by the birth trauma.

Chapter 5. Birth Trauma – Mother

"Giving birth should be your greatest achievement not your greatest fear." – Jane Weideman

Birth trauma can be considered an event that occurs during any phase of the childbearing process that involves actual or threatened serious injury or death to the mother or her infant. The trauma can be classified as a negative outcome, such as postpartum hemorrhage or psychological distress. Experiencing this extremely traumatic stressor, a woman's response can be intense fear, helplessness, loss of control, and horror (Beck, 2004).

Although medicated deliveries are becoming more common, there are considerable adverse circumstances that can influence the mother's breastfeeding abilities, leading to frustration for both mother and baby. For the new mother, increased fluid volume, which is necessary for epidurals due to the risk of hypotension, may cause breast, nipple, or areola edema on the second or third day postpartum. It is this edema that can significantly interfere with baby's capability to latch deeply to the breast and transfer colostrum effectively. Additional fluids can increase the discomfort of lactogenesis II, or copious milk production. Engorgement may follow, which can interfere with successful, comfortable breastfeeding in the first few days at home. Not only does epidural anesthesia impact the baby's ability at the breast, it has been shown to increase intravenous fluid (IV) intake which may effect maternal breast tissue, causing breast edema and making a deep, comfortable latch challenging. Over hydration by IV fluids may result in breast edema, which can cause latch and breast problems (Smith, 2007). A latch made shallow by increased fluid in the breast tissue can cause pain and possible nipple damage for the mother and inadequate milk transfer for the baby. It is possible that administration of IV fluids during labor, which is more prevalent among women who have chosen to receive pain medication, increases the hydration status of the newborn, subsequently leading to the possibility of greater weight loss in the early postpartum period. Degree of weight loss is critical in the decision to supplement breastfed infants (Martens & Romphf, 2007). Epidural use has been associated with delayed and diminished neonatal suckling, and intravenous therapy during labor and delivery may be associated with greater weight loss (Martens & Romphf, 2007), thus resulting in increased risk of supplementation. Formula supplementation of breastfeeding has been consistently associated with shortened breastfeeding duration. Women who use formula supplements in the early postpartum period tend to breastfeed for a shorter time than women who do not supplement (Kurinij & Shiono, 1991).

> Increased fluid volume from medicated births may cause breast, nipple, or areola edema, which interferes with a baby's ability to latch deeply. Increased fluid volume affects the hydration status of the baby, leading to a possible greater weight loss in the early days. Both may result in an increased risk of formula supplementation and shortened breastfeeding duration.

Pitocin, or synthetic oxytocin, is a popular drug used for inducing or augmenting labor by increasing uterine contractions. Oxytocin may also act as an antidiuretic, which can cause additional fluid retention for the mother. A study completed by Jonas, Nissen, Ransjo-Arvidson, Matthiesen, and Uvnas-Moberg (2008) argues that epidural analgesia may block the natural oxytocin release during birth. Some studies show that women having received epidural analgesia have lower circulating oxytocin levels during labor. Jonas et al. (2008) note that women receiving epidural anesthesia received anesthetic bupivacaine in combination with sufentanil for pain relief. The findings in this study are significant due to the importance of oxytocin during labor, delivery, and breastfeeding, encouraging the mother/baby bond after delivery. Delay in this imperative psychological event may lead to decreased breastfeeding and possible supplementation.

> Pitocin may block natural oxytocin release during birth impacting mother/baby bonding after delivery.

In a larger study, Jordan et al. (2009) look at the Cardiff Birth Survey, which includes over 48,000 women. The researchers focused their study on the use of intramuscular oxytocin, having already identified that there is a relationship between epidural fentanyl and lack of breastfeeding. They theorized that up to 200,000 children in the United States would benefit from continued breastfeeding if women were able to avoid medications during labor (2009).

Handlin et al. (2009) examined the effects of sucking, skin-to-skin contact, and stress hormones when influenced by oxytocin and the use of epidural anesthesia. In this study, researchers looked at adrenocorticotropic hormone (ACTH) and cortisol levels, and how epidural anesthesia and oxytocin, either administered intravenously or by injection, may impede breastfeeding. The purpose of ACTH is to regulate cortisol levels. High levels of cortisol have been related to stress, and lower levels with relaxation (2009). The researchers concluded that the more oxytocin the mother received during labor, the lower her circulating oxytocin levels in response to breastfeeding two days postpartum (2009). It was suggested that feedback inhibition of oxytocin release is a reaction to the unphysiological oxytocin levels resulting from oxytocin infusions during labor (2009). Women were exposed to different medical interventions, including epidural anesthesia for pain relief, oxytocin infusion to promote contractions, and oxytocin by injection to prevent postpartum hemorrhage. Handlin et al. noted that ACTH and cortisol levels, after an initial rise, fell significantly during breastfeeding for all women; however, women who received epidural anesthesia in combination with oxytocin experienced higher cortisol levels than women who received only epidural anesthesia (2009). Skin-to-skin contact was associated with lower cortisol levels. Researchers found that oxytocin received by intramuscular injection postpartum facilitated the decrease of cortisol levels caused by skin-to-skin contact (Handlin et al., 2009). Women with oxytocin infusion continued to experience higher cortisol levels. The researchers found that the longer the baby sucked at the breast, the lower the ACTH levels, and the longer the skin-to-skin contact before suckling, the lower the cortisol levels.

> Epidural anesthesia and oxytocin administration during labor increase ACTH and cortisol levels. Skin-to-skin contact and breastfeeding cause ACTH and cortisol levels to fall.

Oxytocin plays a role in the relationship and initial bonding of mother and baby. Women receiving epidural anesthesia have lower levels of oxytocin. Could this possibly impact the brain's ability to make the needed connection between mother and baby in the immediate postpartum period? The mother/baby dyad's capability to touch, smell, and imprint connection after birth have a direct correlation to bonding and baby's self regulation.

There is one unwavering factor to consider when researching breastfeeding initiation and duration. Support for the mother/baby dyad after delivery and after hospital discharge has proven to positively impact breastfeeding initiation and duration, regardless of any intervention the mother may have experienced.

Support

One of the largest variables related to postpartum depression and post-traumatic stress disorder (PTSD) after childbirth is low partner support. In addition to low partner support, high levels of obstetric intervention has been considered to be a risk factor for PTSD after delivery. During labor, women have little to say about what happens to them, and medical decisions may be made without their input. This is especially likely in an emergency. This lack of control can lead to a negative reaction to birth (Kendall-Tackett, 2005).

Three variables related to postpartum depression have been identified as a perceived lack of support during labor and delivery, a high degree of postpartum pain, and a less-than-optimal first contact with their baby (Kendall-Tackett, 2005). All of these traumas can alter a woman's interest and decision to breastfeed. Dissociation due to a traumatized labor, physical pain, and emotional distress not only impacts the physical act of breastfeeding, but also the physiological transformation the body must endure for lactogenesis to be successful. A study done by Beck (2004) recognized that women with severe PTSD symptoms after childbirth experience anxiety attributable to thoughts of the trauma, anger, and emotional detachment from their partners and baby. In addition, Beck, Gable, Sakala, and Declerq (2011) concluded that women who did not breastfeed as long as they wanted or who did not breastfeed exclusively at one-month postpartum had significantly higher PTSD symptom scores. Mothers who recognized that they were traumatized by childbirth shared that flashbacks, disturbing detachment, enduring physical pain, feelings of violation, and insufficient milk supply hindered their breastfeeding attempts (Beck & Watson, 2008). It is difficult to differentiate whether postpartum depression or PTSD leads the mother to abandon breastfeeding, or if it is failure to breastfeed that leads to postpartum depression or PTSD.

> Low partner support and high levels of obstetric intervention during labor and delivery can lead to post-traumatic stress disorder and low breastfeeding rates.

Mimi and Ethan

Mimi had worked in the area of maternal child health for several years and was educated in the field of labor and delivery. She was pregnant with her fourth baby. She expressed concern because although she had always been dedicated to breastfeeding, she knew that her struggles with postpartum depression could be overwhelming. Her last baby was a girl, and Mimi was now expecting a boy. Mimi had always given birth vaginally, but her midwife had discussed with Mimi the possibility of a cesarean delivery due to some underlying complications that might have made vaginal delivery more difficult. When she went into labor, Mimi couldn't help but feel concern regarding her delivery. After Mimi had been laboring for quite a while, the midwife discovered that the umbilical cord had prolapsed and Mimi was rushed in for an emergency cesarean delivery. After her son was delivered, Mimi suffered a severe hemorrhage and lost over half of her natural blood supply.

Because of her medical background, Mimi was aware of what was happening and was convinced that she was going to die before she ever saw her baby.

Since she experienced complications, Mimi was admitted to the Intensive Care Unit of the hospital, and did not receive the same attention and care that a new mother would normally receive. Mimi did not see a lactation consultant while she was in ICU, and she was very concerned about the blood loss affecting her potential milk supply. Mimi did not see her doctor again after her hemorrhage, and she discharged after just a couple of days.

Once home, I went to see Mimi to offer support and to make sure she was doing what she could to encourage a healthy milk supply, despite all that had happened. Ethan was latching well, but Mimi was several days postpartum at this point and her milk was just slowly making an appearance.

"I haven't been able to sleep at all," Mimi confided when I walked in. She had been trying to take a nap before I arrived. "Every time I close my eyes I am afraid I won't wake up. Dianne, I almost died. I knew what was happening. No one really came to check on me after, either. Now I am so afraid that I could develop a blood clot or something, and I will be dead within the week."

There was not much I could say, and not much needed to be said. At this point, the shock was still clearly evident. I did my best to reassure Mimi that she could still develop the relationship with her baby that she desired, and together we created a plan to stimulate her milk supply, while Ethan was fed with donor milk. Because of the blood loss and trauma that Mimi experienced, her milk was delayed, but it was coming in, little by little. Mimi had solid support from family and friends, and was able to slowly recover, however, not without more problems. An infection in her incision left Mimi feeling physically worn out and emotionally drained, with antibiotics leading to thrush for both her and Ethan by the time Ethan was three weeks old. Several months later, Mimi and Ethan were doing wonderfully, and credited much of their success to support that was received during a most difficult time.

Physical or emotional trauma can leave women feeling violated or stripped of their dignity. As a result, some women became vigilant about protecting their bodies, specifically their breasts. It was more important for these women to gain control of their body, and breastfeeding was pushed aside (Beck & Watson, 2008). A woman who feels disappointment or failure about her baby's delivery may reconsider breastfeeding for fear that they will not be successful. Surgical interventions, such as episiotomy and cesarean deliveries, have been linked to breastfeeding difficulties. Episiotomies and third or fourth degree lacerations can cause substantial pain and discomfort for a new mother as she tries to find a comfortable position to feed the baby.

Janine

I was working as an inpatient lactation consultant at a busy hospital. I went in to see Janine, one of the new, first-time mothers who had delivered overnight. I knocked, entered, and introduced myself as the lactation consultant. I asked how breastfeeding was going, and if there were any questions or concerns about the feeds.

"This didn't go how I had planned." These were the first words Janine spoke to me, looking visibly defeated. She was sitting in the bed. "The labor was long, it took longer to push him out than I thought," she waved her hand in the baby's direction, "and I tore pretty bad. I can barely sit down".

I lowered myself into a chair opposite the bed so that I could be face-to-face with Janine. I chose my words carefully. "You have every right to mourn that Janine." She nodded her head. I assisted with helping her latch the baby by letting her stay in bed in a reclined position, with her knees bent and a pillow under them for support. In this position, she was able to take the pressure off her bottom and her son was able to feed in a way that both mom and baby were comfortable.

A study done by Nissen, Gustavsson, Widstrom, and Uvnas-Moberg (1998) found that compared with women who had vaginal births, mothers with cesarean deliveries had a less pulsatile oxytocin-release pattern and lower levels of prolactin, which is critical for successful breastfeeding. Delayed lactogenesis is reported in cesarean deliveries. Women delivering by C-section are more likely to have delayed initial breastfeeding and later onset of lactation; babies have decreased neurological response and are more likely to stop breastfeeding at two weeks (Samuels, Margen, & Schoen, 1985). Women who choose to deliver by elective cesarean section have been found to have higher PTSD symptom scores than those who delivered vaginally or by emergency cesarean delivery. This may be due to fear of childbirth itself, which is why some women elect to deliver by C-section (Keogh, Ayers, & Francis, 2002).

Premature birth can potentially traumatize a new mother, causing detachment from her baby and failed attempts to breastfeed. Admission to a neonatal intensive care unit (NICU) and mother/baby separation play a large role in breastfeeding difficulties. Physical variables, such as birth weight, gestational age, sucking ability, and blood glucose levels, can also impact a baby's ability to exclusively breastfeed, and may increase the need for supplementation by hospital standards. Depending on baby's gestational age and health issues, several days of separation for mother and baby will interfere with a mother's ability to successfully establish an adequate milk supply, which will increase the need for formula supplementation. A new mother may find it difficult to bond with her newborn in the NICU, she may not be able to hold her baby as much as she would like, and she may feel that somehow her body has failed her by not carrying the baby to term.

A preterm birth may impair a mother's ability to bond with her baby.

Rachel – babies Mason and Christopher

Rachel had Mason four years ago. Mason was six weeks premature and never really latched at the breast. Mason had jaundice and was in the NICU for a couple of weeks. Rachel had a history of hormonal complications, which caused an oversupply problem. She attempted to pump for Mason since he wouldn't latch, but developed mastitis four times and switched to formula. Rachel did not feel like she received the breastfeeding help she needed to continue.

Rachel became pregnant with her second baby, who was also born six weeks premature. Rachel's water broke and she was hospitalized for a week before she finally gave birth to Christopher. Rachel had signed up for a breastfeeding class, but went into labor before she could attend. Christopher was also in the NICU for the first couple of weeks, and struggled with jaundice. Rachel once again attempted to breastfeed and pump, more aware of her potential to produce more than the average amount of milk. She found her oversupply difficult to manage while pumping. Rachel called me to help advise her during this difficult time, and confided that with Mason being just four years old, she would not be able to handle the pumping and mastitis that occurred the first time around. Rachel weaned a few weeks after she brought Christopher home.

Both of Rachel's babies were born premature, spent time in the NICU, and developed jaundice. Rachel did not have the opportunity to bond with her babies, hold them when she wanted, and feed them on demand. As noted by Flacking, Ewald, Nyqvist, and Starrin (2006), mothers of preterm or ill infants are most often separated from their infants immediately after birth and during the hospital stay, and the clinical practice can be perceived as task-oriented and focused only on the physical needs of the infant. Infant illness, concern about the outcome, lack of information, poor family functioning, and lack of social support add negatively to the maternal attainment process, causing mothers to experience more stress, depressive symptoms, decreased self-esteem, and impaired later attachment (Flacking et al., 2006). Rachel's breastfeeding experience may have been more positive if she had been able to have more control over the situation after her babies were born.

When working with a mother who has suffered birth trauma, caregivers can be especially helpful in this period by providing the opportunity to discuss the mother's feelings about how the birth transpired and her thoughts and feelings about breastfeeding (Klaus, 2010). In a similar manner to preparing for labor, by listening carefully and validating her feelings in an accepting and nonjudgmental manner, medical personnel and support persons can help the mother explore what concerns she might have and then explore potential solutions (Klaus, 2010). Watching for signs of trauma, including being withdrawn or failing to bond with her infant, can be indicative of a woman struggling to process a traumatic birth. When observing breastfeeding, providers, including hospital lactation consultants, should note if a new mother seems detached from her infant. Not only can birth trauma affect the mother, it can affect her ability to bond with her newborn baby (Callahan & Borja, 2008). It is suggested that clinicians use a tool, such as the Perinatal PTSD Questionnaire, to assist with addressing traumatic birth. Depending on the outcome, this tool can be used to determine if a new mother should be referred for additional help during the postpartum period (Lippincott et al., 2008).

Mary Beth is a very experienced doula. She is well known with providers and trusted among her clients. Mary Beth referred one of her new mothers to me who was struggling with painful feedings in the first few days postpartum. Part of obtaining a thorough history is asking about labor and delivery, since this can be a factor in breastfeeding problems. Together, Mary Beth and Denise described the labor and delivery. Denise recalled lying on her back to push, at the care provider's request. She was pulling her knees up in the typical pushing position and the baby was moving down fairly quickly. She was very trusting of the care provider, even though it was not her chosen doc, and wanted to do what was suggested. Mary Beth mentioned staying in an all fours position, but the nurse said this was how the doc would want her. "I was helping her hold her leg, and Dad was up by mom's head," Mary Beth said. Doc came in and after a few minutes said, "I'm JUST going to give you a little numbing medication on the perineum - nothing else." Denise said ok. " I wasn't sure what his thought was, but recently had a doc recommend that just for mom's sake in case of a tear, so didn't question too much. It had been SO long since I'd seen an episiotomy," Mary Beth stated. "Doc kept looking at me and dad, and finally said, 'Dad, how about you come down here and help catch?' I moved from the position holding her leg and went up to be by mom's head. Dad moved to get gloves on, and I think a nurse came to support her leg. Within just a moment, I heard the episiotomy before I even saw the instrument being taken away. Doc never mentioned it, never asked, never explained. There was no rush, no baby distress, and the head was barely crowning. At first, Denise didn't even know what happened. I heard that haunting sound for days afterward - skin being sliced with scissors."

Denise struggled with finding a comfortable breastfeeding position, and found that sitting in a chair was quite painful for several weeks after delivery.

> Caregivers should watch for signs of a mother failing to bond with her infant. This can indicate the mother's struggle to process a traumatic birth. Allowing a mother to talk about her birth and validating her feelings can help a mother process her trauma and find solutions. Some mothers may need to be referred for additional help during the postpartum period.

Summary

Like birth trauma suffered by the baby, birth trauma suffered by the mother can be easily overlooked. A woman who is devastated by the events of labor and delivery may struggle to initiate a bond with her newborn baby, making breastfeeding difficult.

Symptoms of PTSD related to childbirth are becoming more recognized and identified as a reason why women may abandon breastfeeding earlier. Women have associated lack of support, either by medical personnel or their partner, to be one of the biggest contributors to birth trauma.

Pain suffered in the postpartum period and separation from baby may interfere with a new mother's decision or dedication to breastfeed. Premature delivery can cause a mother to feel detached from her newborn baby and disappointed in how her pregnancy ended. Trying to initiate breastfeeding in a suboptimal environment, such as the NICU, can prove to be discouraging, prompting a new mother to breastfeed less.

Listening to the concerns of a new mother, acknowledging that she is trying to overcome the disappointment of her labor and the delivery of her baby, and offering support may help her to overcome feelings of grief.

Physical trauma, such as pain from an episiotomy or C-section delivery, can be a distraction to a woman who is attempting to initiate breastfeeding. Assisting this mother to position her baby in a way that can be comfortable to both mother and baby will help the mother feel more confident in her breastfeeding ability in the early days.

As with birth trauma that has impacted the baby, it is important for the provider or healthcare worker to be familiar with the mother's history and the history of the labor and delivery. Women who are interested in discussing their trauma should be encouraged to do so. Referrals to programs or individuals who are skilled in working with birth trauma can help to combat depression in the postpartum period.

Chapter 6. Ethics

"Ethics is knowing the difference between what you have a right to do and what is right to do." – Potter Stewart

Ethical Responsibility

Lactation and maternal child health follows the practice of the Universal Principles of Biomedical Ethics, as would any medical organization. It is the ethical responsibility of any provider to offer the best possible care to families, regardless of what the situation is. Looking at how these ethics correlate to breastfeeding and trauma may be helpful to those working closely with new mothers.

Autonomy

Autonomy is the ethical principle that is defined as personal determination, the right of the patient to participate in and finally decide questions involving their care (Edge & Groves, 1998). There are three basic fundamental properties to autonomy. The first of these properties is the ability to decide, the second property is the power to act upon your decision, and, the third property is respecting the autonomy of others. The different traumas that have been discussed in the previous chapters and the outcome of breastfeeding and the new mother are strongly related. In the situation of birth trauma and breastfeeding, studies show that the decision about infant feeding directly relates back to trauma experienced at birth. Many times the decision is made to breastfeed prenatally, but enduring a traumatic labor and delivery may make it impossible for a woman to act upon this decision. It is the responsibility of the health professional under the ethical practice of autonomy to respect any decision that is made by the patient, and to respect her ability to make that decision without judgment.

> Autonomy – the mother's right to make decisions about how best to feed her baby. Caregivers should respect decisions made by the mother without judgment.

Veracity

Veracity is defined as truth telling. The practice of health care is best served in a relationship of trust, where practitioner and patient are bound to the truth (Edge & Groves, 1998). With veracity, trust and honesty between patient and provider are important in following the guideline of this ethical principle. Veracity connects with breastfeeding and trauma in several ways. A provider earning the trust of the patient will promote the honesty needed that will help ensure the best care possible. In the case of sexual abuse and intimate partner violence, a woman may find it difficult to be forthright and honest about abuse that is happening now or has happened in the past. Afraid of being judged and embarrassed of the situation, if there is no trust between patient and provider, the patient may not be honest about the abuse. This will make it complicated for a provider to advise the best practice of care. This may skew information that is passed between provider and patient, including important educational opportunities that may arise. With birth trauma, again the relationship between patient and provider is important, so the patient can feel safe in confiding her feelings and experiences with her provider. The truth may not always be easy to convey between patient and provider, but it is the stepping-stone of the relationship between them.

> Veracity or truth telling between provider and patient is important in providing the best care for mom and baby.

Beneficence

Beneficence is described as the principle that imposes upon the practitioner to seek good for the patient under all circumstances (Edge & Groves, 1998). Beneficence may be a difficult principle to employ, especially if the principle of veracity is not in place. In the situation of breastfeeding and trauma, lack of honesty and trust between practitioner and provider will make it challenging for the provider to seek the best care for the patient. With breastfeeding and sexual abuse, if a patient does not trust her provider enough to be honest about her past, the provider may try to impose the act of breastfeeding upon this mother, with the intent of doing what is best. In actuality, the best thing for this patient would be to find a provider who is skilled in handing sexual abuse survivors. The provider would not be practicing beneficence or what is good for the patient if the truth was unknown. When a provider is aware of the history of his patient, but still does not advise what is for the good of the patient, they would be breaching the Universal Principles of Biomedical Ethics.

> Beneficence is providing the best care for the patient under all circumstances. To do so, the caregiver must be aware of the patient's history.

Janet

Janet attended the healthy pregnancy classes I was facilitating at a community outreach program. Janet was outspoken and forthright, often upsetting other participants with her comments. This was the first baby she had carried to term.

Janet was much easier to handle in a small group setting, or better yet, in a private consultation. Janet was open about her abusive history. The father of her baby was not actively involved, and she was battling his mother and her accusations regarding paternity on an almost daily basis.

One afternoon Janet asked to meet privately with me to formulate a birth plan. Together, Janet and I created a birth plan that was not demanding, but that focused on making her comfortable, considering the abuse in her past. Her birth plan included such things as asking for hospital personnel to knock before entering, wearing her own clothes during labor, and being aware of any procedures that needed to be done.

Janet was receiving care from a clinic that included midwives and she was more receptive and comfortable with female providers. Since Janet was such an advocate for her own care, I encouraged her to make sure her providers were aware of this request.

One afternoon, Janet went for a tour of the hospital where she was to deliver her baby. While on the tour, Janet told the nurse that because of her history of sexual abuse, she was only comfortable working with female providers. "Well, it will just depend on who is on call that day," the nurse responded. This left Janet anxious, afraid, and feeling helpless about labor and delivery. Knowing Janet as I did, she was left to feel defensive. Her fear transformed her into being a demanding and difficult patient.

In a situation such as Janet's, the nurse that was addressing her needs could have encouraged Janet to speak with her provider directly. When Janet disclosed her abuse history and the nurse was not encouraging the best possible care, she was breaching the ethical responsibility of beneficence.

Nonmalfeasance

Nonmalfeasance is defined as the principle that imposes the duty to avoid or refrain from harming the patient. The practitioner who cannot bring about good for the patient is bound by the duty to at least avoid harm (Edge & Groves, 1998). Relating to breastfeeding and trauma, nonmalfeasance protects the patient from harm. In the topic of birth trauma, a new mother may already be suffering from pain inflicted by the birth. An episiotomy would be a good example of pain that a mother may be struggling with. A provider must practice nonmalfeasance when dealing with this patient. It may not be the opinion of the provider to advise against breastfeeding if the mother is experiencing pain, but providers are bound by ethics to support the good of the patient. In a situation such as this, it may be possible for the provider to assist the mother in finding a way to preserve breastfeeding so that she can have time to heal. This principle would go hand-in-hand with autonomy and encouraging the patient to become active in her care. A patient should be made aware of her options and given the opportunity to decide what is best for her.

> Nonmalfeasance – do no harm. Caregivers should make the mother aware of her options and let her decide what is best for her.

Role Fidelity

Role fidelity is another of the Universal Principles of Biomedical Ethics. Role fidelity is the faithful practice of the duties contained in the particular practice (Edge & Groves, 1998). An example of role fidelity as it correlates to breastfeeding and trauma would be if a lactation consultant were to prescribe or recommend a treatment for a mother who had experienced physical harm during her labor with the intent of helping her breastfeed. The lactation consultant might have the best interest of the patient in mind, but by not referring the mother to the appropriate provider, she is not following the Universal Principles of Biomedical Ethics. Role fidelity is when a provider steps outside their scope of practice, therefore resulting in a breach of ethics. By working against role fidelity, a provider is denying the patient the opportunity to reach her goals via a provider who is more skilled in a particular area of expertise. It has been my experience that role fidelity is something that many new breastfeeding mothers fall victim to, because lactation is such an intricate matter, involving both emotional and physical qualities.

> Role fidelity is providing care within your scope of practice and referring appropriately when a situation is outside your scope of practice.

Confidentiality

Confidentiality is defined as the principle that binds the practitioner to hold in strict confidence those things learned about a patient in the course of medical practice (Edge & Groves, 1998). Confidentiality, breastfeeding, and trauma can be connected in a number of ways. A woman may trust her lactation consultant or her provider enough to disclose her history of abuse or to confess current abuse. A woman may do this for several reasons. She may choose to confide in the provider because she wants to receive help, because she wants to talk with someone about her pain, or because she wants to explain why she may choose to discontinue breastfeeding. Whatever the reason, if a provider does not keep this information private, they are breaching the confidentiality of the patient. This is a serious offense. In violating this ethical principle, a provider is also breaching the other ethical principles. The Universal Principles of Biomedical Ethics that have been defined thus far all have an element of confidentiality that should be followed. Breaching this important principle not only destroys the relationship between patient and provider, it may damage any future relationship that this patient attempts to facilitate with another provider.

> Confidentiality means not discussing information a client has shared with anyone else, unless given permission by the client.

Justice

The final principle in the Universal Principles of Biomedical Ethics, justice is defined as the basic principle that deals with fairness, just desserts, and entitlement in the distribution of goods and service (Edge & Groves, 1998). In all aspects of healthcare, and especially in maternal child health and lactation, this is an important principle to follow. It seems that in healthcare, justice is not always preserved, and those that are more affluent have the best care, best providers, and best medication. Justice relates to the subject of breastfeeding and trauma in this way. As mentioned in the previous section, studies show that women who are victims of sexual abuse, childhood sexual abuse, or domestic violence are more likely to be from lower socioeconomic status, have lower education levels, and may engage in habits, such as smoking and drug abuse. Should these victimized women receive a lower level of care? A provider is responsible for ensuring justice and equality within their scope of practice.

We have discussed that women who are more likely to have suffered abuse or who are at higher risk for abuse are women who live in poverty and who have been exposed to a lower level of education. These women are residing in communities where it is more difficult to find good healthcare, have fewer options for healthcare, and are limited by insurance. The clinics where they go for medical care might be crowded, which leaves little time for a provider to educate their patient and foster an appropriate relationship. By finding ways to connect with the patient and ensuring that they are receiving the attention that is needed, providers can exercise justice by making sure that they are spending time with patients and suggesting community programs and outreach activities that will help to educate and empower a new mother.

> Justice means providing the best care for every client, regardless of background, income level, or any other variable.

Summary

The medical profession, including the field of maternal child health and lactation, follows the Universal Principles of Biomedical Ethics. These ethical principles, which incorporate autonomy, veracity, beneficence, nonmalfeasance, role fidelity, confidentiality, and justice, play an important role in how a provider should support a new mother.

Each of these significant principles relate to breastfeeding and trauma in its own way, prompting how a provider might interact with a new mother and impacting decisions that they might make during this delicate period. Providers should pay particular attention to respecting the confidentiality of the patient and knowing when to refer a patient to someone who may be more familiar with a difficult situation.

Chapter 7. Conclusion

For decades, women have been breastfeeding their babies. Formula was not introduced until almost the 20th century. More and more women began using breastmilk substitutes, and by the 1970s, breastfeeding had decreased significantly. With this increased acceptance of human milk substitutes as convenient and "scientific," breastfeeding rates began to steadily drop. Initiation rates in the United States reached an all-time low of 24.7% in 1971, with less than 10% of mothers continuing as long as three months (Martinez & Nalenzienski, 1979).

Breastfeeding is again on the rise in the 21st century. Medical professionals are recognizing the fascinating elements of breastfeeding for mother and baby. With the Baby Friendly Hospital Initiative becoming more desirable, continued guidance from the Joint Commission, and the inclusion of breastfeeding support in the workplace and the Healthcare Reform, breastfeeding goals are becoming more attainable. Even with all the evidence-based research and verification from healthcare professionals, there are still some strong barriers to breastfeeding. In my work as a lactation consultant, I have seen barriers to breastfeeding that can be difficult to conquer. The examples of sexual abuse, intimate partner violence, and birth trauma that have filled the pages of this book have been real situations that I have experienced. I have been fortunate to be part of the lives of so many mothers who were willing to come face-to-face with their trauma in order to nurture a breastfeeding relationship with their baby.

With sexual abuse and intimate partner violence, women can be reluctant to disclose their abusive past. This may be due to embarrassment, fear of being judged, fear of their abuser, or distrust of their healthcare provider. Regardless of what the reason is, the relationship with their newborn baby may be effected by their past experiences.

Women struggling with birth trauma may also struggle with the internal conflict that can arise when their trauma has been minimized. A woman intending to have a vaginal birth and who delivers via C-section may repress feelings of disappointment because she is told she should be grateful her baby was born healthy. Resentment may follow, resentment towards the delivery, her body, and her support system can spiral downward, making bonding and breastfeeding almost impossible.

It is not a guarantee that women who have experienced sexual abuse in childhood will abandon breastfeeding. Many survivors will initiate breastfeeding with the best of intentions. However, sometimes unresolved feelings can be pushed too far, causing the new mother to wean her baby earlier than intended. In other circumstances, breastfeeding can be an amazing experience for the abuse survivor, empowering her ability to care for her baby and reclaim her sense of self.

The topic of breastfeeding and trauma is a subject that does not discriminate. It can be recognized in all areas of the world in many ways. Some areas of humankind may be more prone to abuse than birth trauma, and some may see more domestic violence than sexual abuse.

The Population Information Program and the Center for Gender Equity, two respected research institutions based in Washington, D.C., studied numerous local research projects and produced findings in 1999 that echo the consensus of numerous public health and human rights authorities: around the world, at least one woman in every three has been coerced into sex, or otherwise beaten in her lifetime (Murray, 2008). Potentially, abuse, birth trauma, and resistance to breastfeeding can all happen under the same umbrella. In situations of domestic or sexual abuse, forced intercourse may cause pregnancy. In countries where there is conflict, sexual abuse against women is a form of combat. Militarized rape, particularly the version that uses forced pregnancy as a kind of biological warfare was used widely by the Yugoslav Army, the Bosnian Serb forces, and the irregular Serb militia as part of the Serbian genocidal policy of "ethnic cleansing" and "cultural cleansing" during the conflict (Murray, 2008). Such trauma before and during pregnancy can undoubtedly cause birth trauma during labor and delivery for a woman who was forcibly impregnated. Dissociation and detachment would lead this mother to feelings of hostility and regret towards her child. Would a woman who had endured such a hardship be able to sustain the intimate and nurturing relationship that breastfeeding demands?

Birth trauma that is suffered by mother, baby, or both can also be a difficult hurdle to overcome. Many women prepare for childbirth by taking classes and learning all they can about how to have the so-called "perfect birth." Many women have a picture in their head of how they are expecting the birth of their baby to occur, and if this goes awry, feelings of anguish may take over. Post-traumatic stress disorder is becoming more recognized among women after childbirth, and to these women breastfeeding may not seem as important anymore as it once was. Health professionals should acknowledge that a new mother might need time to grieve a delivery that did not go as planned. Physical trauma for the baby may be harder to recognize, and healthcare professionals should be aware that long labors, Cesarean births, and operative deliveries may lead to feeding difficulties for a newborn baby. Of course, not every baby born by cesarean delivery will struggle with feeding or positional problems during a feeding, but being aware that this may be the answer if difficulties occur is an important piece to troubleshooting breastfeeding problems.

My work with breastfeeding mothers from different demographics has been vast. In all areas, I have found that all new mothers want what is best for their baby, but some mothers are unsure of how to make this happen or do not have the support to make this happen. All new mothers want to be the best mother they can be. In many situations, these mothers have endured abuse that is unimaginable. Some are willing to learn more about breastfeeding, and some are resistant to the intimacy that breastfeeding brings. While researching breastfeeding and trauma, I have learned how important it is to be respectful and nonjudgmental when dealing with a new mother who is struggling with aspects of breastfeeding and trauma. Often I have heard women voice their frustration when dealing with a provider who is insensitive or who doesn't take the time to listen to her requests. Asking the new mother questions about how she perceived her labor and delivery is a window into her recovery. Asking a woman her thoughts about breastfeeding in the prenatal period can be a strong indicator of whether or not there is a history of abuse. The nurturing bond, health benefits, and empowerment that a woman can experience while breastfeeding is particularly powerful for any woman. However, it is important to remember that every mother is not able to get past her feelings and accept a healthy breastfeeding relationship with her baby. As a lactation consultant, it is imperative to acknowledge limits and recognize what she is willing to give. Being able to recognize signs of abuse in a new mother or signs of birth trauma in a newborn baby can make a difference in whether or not a woman pursues a breastfeeding relationship with her baby. This is an often-overlooked yet important part of supporting a new mother.

Realizing that a new mother may not be able to get past her trauma or abuse is a concept that may be difficult for providers or lactation consultants. Becoming familiar with the patient's history is the first step in being able to offer viable solutions and suggestions. Including the new mother in the decision-making process and making a plan together will help to empower a new mother and help her feel supported. By offering a nonjudgmental attitude towards a new mother, she will be more likely to disclose her concerns. Women who feel supported during the prenatal and postpartum period are more likely to breastfeed for a longer period of time.

Working with women who have endured abuse and trauma is never easy. It is critical to remember that trauma affects everyone differently. Put aside any personal feelings and concentrate on what will help the mother/baby dyad. Sometimes the solution is to stop breastfeeding altogether, and encouraging pumping breastmilk and close bonding. Sometimes the solution is keeping the new mother engaged in constant support and encouragement, which can be exhausting for the provider. Realizing limits and boundaries is fundamental. Working with women who have endured abuse and trauma can also be very rewarding. It is inspiring to see a mother work through her despair and develop an amazing breastfeeding relationship with her baby.

References

American Pregnancy Association. (2007). *Epidural anesthesia.* Retrieved from http://americanpregnancy.org/labornbirth/epidural.html

Archabald, K., Lundsberg, L., Triche, E., Norwitz, E., & Illuzzi, J. (2011). Women's prenatal concerns regarding breastfeeding: Are they being addressed? *J Midwifery Womens Health, 56*(1), 2-7.

Beck, C.T. (2004). Post traumatic stress disorder due to childbirth: The aftermath. *Nursing Research 53*(4), 216-224.

Beck, C.T., Gable, R.K., Sakala, C., & Declercq, E.R., (2011). Posttraumatic stress disorder in new mothers: Results from a two-stage U.S. national survey. *Birth: Issues in Perinatal Care, (38)* 3, 216-227.

Beck, C., & Watson, S. (2008). Impact of birth trauma on breastfeeding: A tale of two pathways. *Nursing Research, 57*(4), 228-236.

Berry, D. (2006). *Health communication: Theory and practice.* Buckingham, GBR: Open University Press.

Black, M. (2011). Intimate partner violence and adverse health consequences. Implications for clinicians. *American Journal of Lifestyle Medicine, 5*(5), 428-439.

Bowman, K. (2007). When breastfeeding may be a threat to adolescent mothers. *Issues in Mental Health Nursing, 28*, 89-99.

Bowman, K.G., Ryberg, J.W., & Becker, H. (2009). Examining the relationship between a childhood history of sexual abuse and later dissociation, breastfeeding practices and parenting anxiety. *J Interpers Violence, 24*(8), 1304-1317.

Brooks, E.C. (2013). *Legal and ethical issues for the IBCLC.* Burlington, MA: Jones and Bartlett Learning.

Browne, A., & Finkelhor, D. (1986). Impact of child sexual abuse: A review of the research. *Psychol Bull, 99*(1), 66-77.

Bureau of Justice Statistics. (2014). National crime victimization survey. Retrieved from http://www.data.gov/raw/1526/

Callahan, J., & Borja, S. (2008). Psychological outcomes and measurement of maternal post traumatic stress disorder during the perinatal period. *Journal of Perinatal and Neonatal Nursing, 22*(1), 49-59.

CDC (2012). *Breastfeeding among U.S. children born 2000-2010, CDC National Immunization Survey.* Retrieved from http://www.cdc.gov/breastfeeding/data/NIS_data/

CDC. (2014). Intimate partner violence. Retrieved from www.cdc.gov ViolencePrevention/intimatepartnerviolence/index.html

Cerulli, C., Chin, N., Talbot, N., & Chaudron, L. (2010). Exploring the impact of intimate partner violence on breastfeeding initiation: Does it matter? *Journal of Breastfeeding Medicine, 5*(5), 225.

Chen, D.C., Nommsen-Rivers, L., Dewey, K.G., Lonnerdal, B. (1998). Stress during labor and delivery and early lactation performance. *American Journal of Clinical Nutrition, 68*(2), 335-344.

Coles, J., Jones, K. (2009). "Universal precautions:" Perinatal touch and examination after childhood sexual abuse. *Birth, 36*(3), 230-236.

Dewey, K.G. (2001). Maternal and fetal stress are associated with impaired lactogenesis in humans. *Journal of Nutrition, 131*(11), 3012-3015.

Dictionary.com. (2014). Trauma. Retrieved from http://dictionary.reference.com/browse/trauma?s=t

DiLillo, D. (2001). Interpersonal functioning among women reporting a history of childhood sexual abuse: Empirical findings and methodological issues. *Clinical Psychology Review, 21*(4), 553-576.

Douglas, A.R. (2000). Reported anxieties concerning intimate parenting in women sexually abused as children. *Child Abuse & Neglect, 24*, 425-434.

Dubowitz, H., Black, M.M., Kerr, M.A., Hussey, J.M., Morrel, T.M., Everson, M.D., & Starr, Jr., R.H., (2001). Type and timing of mothers' victimization: *Effects of mothers and children. Pediatrics, 107*(4), 728-735.

Edge, R.S., & Groves, J.R. (2007). *Ethics of health care: A guide for clinical practice.* Clifton Park, NY : Thomson Delmar Learning.

English, D.J., Upadhyaya, M.P., Litrownik, A.J., Marshall, J.M., Runyan, D.K., Graham, J., & Dubowitz, H. (2005). Maltreatment's wake: The relationship of maltreatment dimensions to child outcomes. *Child Abuse & Neglect, 29*, 597-619.

Flacking, R., Ewald, U., Nyqvist, K.H., & Starrin, B. (2006). Trustful bonds: A key to "becoming a mother" and to reciprocal breastfeeding. Stories of mothers of very preterm infants at a neonatal unit. *Soc Sci Med, 62*(1), 70-80.

Hall, R.T., Mercer, A.M., Teasley, S.L., McPherson, D.M., Simon, S.D., Santos, S.R., et al. (2002). A breast-feeding assessment score to evaluate the risk for cessation of breast-feeding by 7 to 10 days of age. *The Journal of Pediatrics, 141*(5), 659-64.

Handlin, L., Jonas, W., Petersson, M., Ejdeback, M., Ransjo-Arvidson, A.B., Nissen, E., & Uvnas-Moberg, K. (2009). Effects of sucking and skin-to-skin contact on maternal ACTH and cortisol levels during the second day postpartum-influence of epidural analgesia and oxytocin in the perinatal period. *Breastfeed Med, 4*(4), 207-220.

Henderson, J.J., Dickinson, J.E., Evans, S.F., McDonald, S.J., & Paech, M.J. (2003). Impact of intrapartum epidural analgesia on breast-feeding duration. *Aust N Z J Obstet Gynaecol, 43*(5), 372-277.

Howie, W.O., & McMullen, P.C. (2006). Breastfeeding problems following anesthetic administration. *J Perinat Educ, 15*(3), 50-57.

Jonas, W., Nissen, E., Ransjo-Arvidson, A.B., Matthiesen, A.S., & Uvnas-Moberg, K. (2008). Influence of oxytocin or epidural analgesia on personality profile in breastfeeding women: A comparative study. *Arch Womens Ment Health, 11*(5-6), 335-345.

Jordan, S., Emery, S, Bradshaw, Watkins, & Friswell, W. (2005). The impact of intrapartum analgesia on infant feeding. *BJOG, 112*(7), 927-934.

Jordan, S., Emery, S., Watkins, A., Evans, J.D., Storey, M., & Morgan, G., (2009). Association of drugs routinely given in labour with breastfeeding at 48 hours: Analysis of the Cardiff Births Survey. *BJOG, 116*(12), 1622-1629.

Karl, D. (2004). Behavioral state organization: Breastfeeding. *MCN: The American Journal of Maternal/Child Nursing, 29*, 293–298.

Kendall-Tackett, K. (Ed.). (2005). *Handbook of women, stress and trauma*. New York, NY: Brunner-Rutledge.

Kendall-Tackett, K.A. (2007). Violence against women in the perinatal period: The Impact of a lifetime of violence and abuse on pregnancy, postpartum and breastfeeding. *Trauma Violence Abuse 2007, (8)* 344.

Keogh, E., Ayers, S., & Francis, H. (2002). Does anxiety sensitivity predict post-traumatic stress symptoms following childbirth? A preliminary report. *Cogn Behav Ther, 31*, 145–155.

Klaus, P. (2010). The impact of childhood sexual abuse on childbearing and breastfeeding: The role of maternity caregivers. *Journal of Breastfeeding Medicine, 5*(4), 141-145.

Kurinij, N., & Shiono, P.H. (1991). Early formula supplementation of breast-feeding. *Pediatrics, 88*(4), 745-750.

Lau, Y., & Chan, K.S. (2007). Influence of intimate partner violence during pregnancy and early postpartum depressive symptoms on breastfeeding among Chinese women in Hong Kong. *Journal of Midwifery & Women's Health, 52*(5), e15-e20.

Lawrence, R.A., & Lawrence, R.M. (2005). *Breastfeeding: A guide for the medical profession.* Philadelphia: Mosby.

Martens, P.J., & Romphf, L. (2007). Factors associated with newborn in-hospital weight loss: Comparisons by feeding method, demographics, and birthing procedures. *J Hum Lact, 23*(3), 233-241.

Martinez, G.A., & Nalenzienski, J.P. (1979). The recent trend in breastfeeding. *Pediatrics, 64,* 686-692.

Mezey, G., Bacchus, L., Bewley, S., & White, S. (2005). Domestic violence, lifetime trauma and psychological health of childbearing women, *BJOG, 112*(2), 197-204.

Murray, S. (2008). Why doesn't she just leave?: Belonging, disruption and domestic violence. *Women's Studies International Forum, 31* (1), 65-72.

Nissen, E., Gustavsson, P., Widstrom, A.M., & Uvnas-Moberg, K. (1998). Oxytocin, prolactin, milk production and their relationship with personality traits in women after vaginal delivery or Cesarean section. *Journal of Psychosomatic Obstretics & Gynecology, 19*(1), 49-58.

Perkins, C., Klaus, P., Bastian, L., and Cohen, R. (1996). Criminal victimization in the United States, 1993: A National Crime Victimization Survey Report. The U.S. Department of Justice Bureau of Justice Statistics. Washington, DC: USGPO

Prentice, J.C., Lu, M.C., Lange, L., & Halfon, N. (2002). The association between reported childhood sexual abuse and breastfeeding initiation. *Journal of Human Lactation, 18*(3), 219-226.

Russell, D.E.A. (1986). *The secret trauma incest in the lives of girls and women.* New York, NY: Basic Books.

Samuels, S.E., Margen, S., Schoen, E.J. (1985). Incidence and duration of breastfeeding in a health maintenance organization population. *American Journal of Clinical Nutrition, 42*(3), 504-510.

Silberg, J., Waters, F., Nemzer, E., McIntee, J., Wieland, S., Grimminck, E., Nordquist, L., & Emsond, E. (2003). Guidelines for the evaluation and treatment of dissociative symptoms in children and adolescents-2003- ISSD Task Force on Children and Adolescents. Retrieved from http://www.isst-d.org/default.asp?contentID=50

Silverman, J.G., Decker, M.R., Reed, E., & Raj, A. (2006). Intimate partner violence around the time of pregnancy: Association with breastfeeding behavior. *Journal of Women's Health, 15*(8), 934-940.

Smith, L. (2010). *Impact of birthing practices on breastfeeding.* Second edition. Sudbury, MA: Jones and Bartlett Publishers.

Stampfel, C.C., Chapman, D.A., & Alvarez, A.E. (2010). Intimate partner violence and posttraumatic stress disorder among high-risk women: Does pregnancy matter? *Violence Against Women, 16*(4), 426-443.

U.S. Department of Health and Human Services, Health Resources and Services Administration, Maternal and Child Health Bureau. (2009). *Child Health USA 2008-2009*. Rockville, Maryland: U.S. Department of Health and Human Services. Retrieved from http://mchb.hrsa.gov/chusa08/hstat/hsi/pages/201b.html

U.S. Department of Health and Human Services, Health Resources and Services Administration, Maternal and Child Health Bureau. (2013). *Child Health USA 2013*. Rockville, Maryland: U.S. Department of Health and Human Services. Retrieved from http://mchb.hrsa.gov/chusa13/perinatal-risk-factors-behaviors/p/breastfeeding.html

Index

About the Author

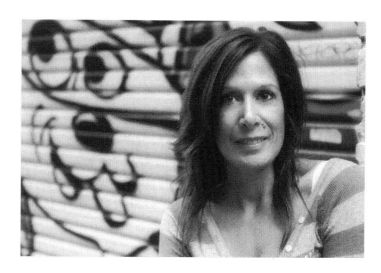

Dianne Cassidy has been working with breastfeeding mothers for eight years in Rochester, New York. Starting out as a WIC Peer Counselor, she became an IBCLC with an advanced certification. She was fortunate to be able to visit mothers in their homes in the city of Rochester, where she first became familiar with how trauma impacts new mothers.

As an IBCLC, Dianne has worked in hospitals, with community outreach pregnancy programs, and in Private Practice. Her work with underprivileged women has led to her research into how trauma in all forms impacts breastfeeding. She began this research while completing her Bachelor of Science degree in Maternal Child Health/Lactation. She received her Master's degree in 2013. The increased awareness she has found for these mothers has made her a better lactation consultant to all mothers.

69248974R00046

Made in the USA
Middletown, DE
19 September 2019